THE TRUTH ABOUT VIOLENCE

THE TRUTH ABOUT VIOLENCE

SECOND EDITION

Robert N. Golden, M.D.
University of Wisconsin–Madison
General Editor

Fred L. Peterson, Ph.D.
University of Texas–Austin
General Editor

Karl Larson, Ph.D., and William McCay
Principal Authors

Heath Dingwell, Ph.D.
Contributing Author

William Kane, Ph.D.
University of New Mexico
Adviser to the First Edition

Mark J. Kittleson, Ph.D.
Southern Illinois University
Adviser to the First Edition

Richelle Rennegarbe, Ph.D.
McKendree College
Adviser

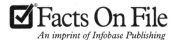

Facts On File
An imprint of Infobase Publishing

The Truth About Violence, Second Edition

Facts On File, Inc.
An imprint of Infobase Publishing
132 West 31st Street
New York NY 10001

Library of Congress Cataloging-in-Publication Data

Larson, Karl.
    The truth about violence / Robert N. Golden, general editor, Fred L. Peterson, general editor; Karl Larson and William McCay, principal authors; Health Dingwell, contributing author; William Kane, adviser to the first edition, Mark J. Kittleson, adviser to the first edition ; Richelle Rennegarbe. – 2nd ed.
      p. cm.
    Includes bibliographical references and index.
    ISBN-13: 978-0-8160-7644-4 (hardcover : alk. paper)
    ISBN-10: 0-8160-7644-8 (hardcover : alk. paper) 1. Violence in adolescence–United States–Juvenile literature. 2. Teenagers–United States–Juvenile literature. I. Dingwell, Heath. II. McCay, William. III. Golden, Robert N. IV. Title.
    HQ799.2.V56L37 2010
    303.60973–dc22   2010000973

Facts On File books are available at special discounts when purchased in bulk quantities for businesses, associations, institutions, or sales promotions. Please call our Special Sales Department in New York at (212) 967-8800 or (800) 322-8755.

You can find Facts On File on the World Wide Web at http://www.factsonfile.com

Text design by David Strelecky
Composition by Mary Susan Ryan-Flynn
Cover printed by Art Print, Taylor, PA
Book printed and bound by Maple Press, York, PA
Date printed: November 2010
Printed in the United States of America

10 9 8 7 6 5 4 3 2 1

This book is printed on acid-free paper.

CONTENTS

List of Illustrations and Tables   vii

Preface   ix

How to Use This Book   xi

Violent Behavior and Personal Safety   1

A–to–Z Entries   **11**

  Alcohol and Violence   13

  Anger Management   17

  Assault and Bullying   22

  Communities and Violence   27

  Criminals and Violent Activity   31

  Drugs and Violence   36

  Family Violence   41

  Fight or Flight Response   48

  Gang Violence   53

  Hate Crimes   61

  Homicide   66

  Incarceration   70

  Intermittent Explosive Disorder   78

  Legal Interventions   85

Media and Violence   90
Rehabilitation and Treatment of Perpetrators   94
Revenge, Cycle of   100
Road Rage   106
School Violence   109
Self-mutilation   116
Sexual Violence   119
Social Costs of Violence   127
Suicide   132
Teens and Violence   137
Terrorism   145
Violence Against Populations   152
Violence and Video Games   158
Violent Behavior, Causes of   164
War   171
Weapons of Violence   176
Workplace Violence   182
Hotlines and Help Sites   189
Glossary   193
Index   201

LIST OF ILLUSTRATIONS

How Anger Can Be Expressed in School   20

Locations of Bullying   24

Estimated Average Time to Be Served
Under Truth-in-Sentencing Laws   33

Persons Raped or Physically Assaulted in
Their Lifetime, by Gender of Victim   46

Stress Sources, As of 2003   49

Risk Factors at Ages 10–12 for Gang Membership   57

People in U.S. Prisons or Jails   71

Prisoner Admissions and Releases, 2000–2006   73

Sentencing Guidelines for the State of Washington   74

Student Suicide Trends in the United States   81

National Rate of Recidivism, Within Three Years,
of State Prisoners Released in 1994, by Prisoner
Characteristics   97

Gang Violence in Los Angeles, February, 2009   102

Students Carrying Weapons on School Grounds,
1993–2005   115

Percentage of High School Students Who Carried
a Gun or Other Weapon, by Ethnicity, Sex, and Grade   142

Terrorism-Related Deaths, by Method of Attack   146

Breaches in Cybersecurity   148

Violence and Hate Crimes   153

Motivation for Hate Crimes   156

Illicit Drug Use Among 12–17-Year-Olds, 2002–2007   168

Firearm-Related Juvenile Homicide Victims,
2002–2007   177

Homicides in the Workplace   182

PREFACE

The Truth About series—updated and expanded to include 20 volumes—seeks to identify the most pressing health issues and social challenges confronting our nation's youth. Adolescence is the period between the onset of puberty and the attainment of adulthood. Adolescence is also a time of storm, stress, and risk-taking for many young people. During adolescence, a person's health is influenced by biological, psychological, and social factors, all of which interact with one's environment—family, peers, school, and community. It is a time when teenagers experience profound changes.

With the latest available statistics and new insights that have emerged from ongoing research, the Truth About series seeks to help young people build a foundation of information as they face some of the challenges that will affect their health and well-being. These challenges include high-risk behaviors, such as drinking, smoking, and other drug use; sexual behaviors that can lead to adolescent pregnancy and sexually transmitted diseases (STDs), such as HIV/AIDS; mental-health concerns, such as depression and suicide; learning disorders and disabilities, which are often associated with school failures and school dropouts; serious family problems, including domestic violence and abuse; and lifestyle factors, which increase adolescents' risk for noncommunicable diseases, such as diabetes and cardiovascular disease, among others.

Broader underlying factors also influence adolescent health. These include socioeconomic circumstances, such as poverty; available health care, and the political and social situations in which young people live. Although these factors can negatively affect adolescent health and well-being, as well as school performance, many of these negative health outcomes are preventable with the proper knowledge and information.

With prevention in mind, the writers and editors of each topical volume in the Truth About series have tried to provide cutting-edge information that is supported by research and scientific evidence. Vital facts are presented that inform youth about the challenges experienced during adolescence, while special features seek to dispel common myths and misconceptions. Some of the main topics explored include abuse, alcohol, death and dying, divorce, drugs, eating disorders, family life, fear and depression, rape, sexual behavior and unplanned pregnancy, smoking, and violence. All volumes discuss risk-taking behaviors and their consequences, healthy choices, prevention, available treatments, and where to get help.

In this new edition of the series, we also have added eight new titles in areas of increasing significance to today's youth. ADHD, or attention-deficit/hyperactivity disorder, and learning disorders are diagnosed with increasing frequency; and many students have observed or know of classmates receiving treatment for these conditions, even if they have not themselves received this diagnosis. Gambling is gaining currency in our culture, as casinos open and expand in many parts of the country, and the Internet offers easy access for this addictive behavior. Another consequence of our increasingly "online" society, unfortunately, is the presence of online predators. Environmental hazards represent yet another danger, and it is important to provide unbiased information about this topic to our youth. Suicide, which for many years has been a "silent epidemic," is now gaining recognition as a major public health problem throughout the life span, including the teenage and young adult years. We now also offer an overview of illness and disease in a volume that includes the major conditions of particular interest and concern to youth. In addition to illness, however, it is essential to emphasize health and its promotion, and this is especially apparent in the volumes on physical fitness and stress management.

It is our intent that each book serve as an accessible, authoritative resource that young people can turn to for accurate and meaningful answers to their specific questions. The series can help them research particular problems and provide an up-to-date evidence base. It is also designed with parents, teachers, and counselors in mind so that they have a reliable resource that they can share with youth who seek their guidance.

Finally, we have tried to provide unbiased facts rather than subjective opinions. Our goal is to help elevate the health of the public with an emphasis on its most precious component—our youth. As young people face the challenges of an increasingly complex world, we as educators want them to be armed with the most powerful weapon available—knowledge.

Robert N. Golden, M.D.
Fred L. Peterson, Ph.D.
General Editors

HOW TO
USE THIS BOOK

NOTE TO STUDENTS

Knowledge is power. By possessing knowledge you have the ability to make decisions, ask follow-up questions, or know where to go to obtain more information. In the world of health that *is* power! That is the purpose of this book—to provide you with the power you need to obtain unbiased, accurate information and *The Truth About Violence.*

Topics in each volume of The Truth About series are arranged in alphabetical order, from A to Z. Each of these entries defines its topic and explains in detail the particular issue. At the end of most entries are cross-references to related topics. A list of all topics by letter can be found in the table of contents or at the back of the book in the index.

How have these books been compiled? First, the publisher worked with me to identify some of the country's leading authorities on key issues in health education. These individuals were asked to identify some of the major concerns that young people have about such topics. The writers read the literature, spoke with health experts, and incorporated their own life and professional experiences to pull together the most up-to-date information on health issues, particularly those of interest to adolescents and of concern in Healthy People 2010.

Throughout the alphabetical entries, the reader will find sidebars that separate Fact from Fiction. There are Question-and-Answer boxes that attempt to address the most common questions that youths ask about sensitive topics. In addition, readers will find a special feature called "Teens Speak"—case studies of teens with personal stories related to the topic in hand.

This may be one of the most important books you will ever read. Please share it with your friends, families, teachers, and classmates. Remember, you possess the power to control your future. One way to affect your course is through the acquisition of knowledge. Good luck and keep healthy.

NOTE TO LIBRARIANS

This book, along with the rest of The Truth About series, serves as a wonderful resource for young researchers. It contains a variety of facts, case studies, and further readings that the reader can use to help answer questions, formulate new questions, or determine where to go to find more information. Even though the topics may be considered delicate by some, do not be afraid to ask patrons if they have questions. Feel free to direct them to the appropriate sources, but do not press them if you encounter reluctance. The best we can do as educators is to let young people know that we are there when they need us.

Mark J. Kittleson, Ph.D.
Adviser to the First Edition

VIOLENT BEHAVIOR AND PERSONAL SAFETY

Violence is the use of force, either in action or behavior, to harm another person. For most people, the word *violence* suggests physical harm, but violence can also result in emotional or mental distress. The concept of violence covers a broad range of behavior. It includes shootings, robbery, sexual assault or rape, child abuse, spousal abuse, and any other form of physical assault on another person. Throughout this book such acts fall under the category of violent crime. There is also the violence that is an integral part of war. And increasingly Americans are experiencing terrorism. A form of violence directed at civilians and political leaders, terrorism is meant to instill fear and to force political change, allowing a small number of people to have a devastating impact on a whole society.

NEW TO THE REVISED EDITION

Even though violence has been declining, according to the latest statistics, it is still a significant problem in the United States. Violence is the second leading cause of death of people between the ages of 10 and 24. Eighty-two percent of homicide victims in this age group were killed with a gun, and there is still a strong relationship between violence and both alcohol and drug use.

In addition to updating the statistics on violence, seven new entries have been added to *The Truth About Violence*. These include anger management, incarceration, intermittent explosive disorder, cycle of revenge, terrorism, violence against populations, and violence and video games.

For decades, there has been an established relationship linking video game violence and violent behavior. Most of the research has shown that the more violent video games a person plays, the more likely that person is to express violent thoughts or actions.

Needless to say, terrorism has become a key issue in the United States since September 11, 2001. Security concerns even dominated the presidential elections in 2004. Terrorism involves violence that is extremely difficult to combat—all it takes is one person, a lone assailant, to commit such an unimaginable act. In this entry, there is also a discussion of cyberterrorism and biological terrorism, two types of terrorism against which the United States is still grappling.

Related to terrorism is violence against populations. This entry focuses on violence against specific groups of people. Hate crimes can be considered a subset of this. Genocide is a large-scale means of violence against groups. This entry examines some of the current examples of genocide, such as the examples of Darfur and Rwanda.

Another entry focuses on intermittent explosive disorder. This is a disorder characterized by aggressive behavior that is out of proportion to circumstances.

The entry on incarceration provides a brief history of U.S. prisons, the different types of prisons, and the goals of prisons. The primary goal of incarceration is simple: to keep offenders away from the public. The prison system is also supposed to act as a deterrent to others who are considering criminal behavior.

Anger management is another new entry to this second edition. There are healthy and unhealthy ways to deal with anger and other negative emotions. When people do not properly express their feelings, conflict can develop with other people. Further, anger has negative effects on the body. People who do not properly deal with their anger can develop or worsen physical conditions, such as pain.

Finally, in the entry on the cycle of revenge, readers will find information on both the motivation behind revenge and retaliation and on intergenerational violence, or the cycle of violence.

FORMS OF VIOLENCE

Violence is not always obvious. Bullying may or may not include physical harm. Creating fear in a classmate is a form of bullying, although the aggressive student may never physically touch his or her victim. Neglect is a form of violence in which not doing something is the crime. Manipulating the feelings of children and intimate partners is a form of violence commonly called emotional abuse. In fact, this type of abuse can create such a fearful environment that daily living becomes a challenge. This book will discuss many forms of violent behavior, their origins, and how they impact individuals and communities.

It seems almost impossible to escape violence these days. Turn on the television news, read a newspaper, click on any news site, or even talk to your friends in the lunchroom, and you'll hear about some sort of violence. Thousands get killed every day in our nation, and many times more suffer injury, humiliation, embarrassment, threats, violation, robbery, or torture. Americans are confronted with so much violence today that many people react to stories about violent acts with a shrug, perhaps suggesting violence seems beyond anyone's control.

A HISTORY OF VIOLENCE

Violence has impacted humanity since before history. Even the earliest human cultures killed in order to eat meat and wear animal skins. Studying the fossil record of North and South America, paleoarcheologists, scientists who examine the remains of prehistoric cultures, found a remarkably efficient spearhead called the Clovis point that was made in North America approximately 15,000 years ago. As scientists tracked the spread of the Clovis point, they noticed that the remains of large mammals like the mammoth and the giant sloth decreased. The animals became extinct—hunted out of existence by people who killed them for sustenance.

As civilization developed, violence did not disappear. For more than 600 years, citizens of Rome filled large arenas to watch gladiators fight to the death. In the 1600s the English theater that produced William Shakespeare's plays was located near a bear-garden. Here, bears would be chained to a post to fight to the death with pairs of dogs. Fans included King Henry VIII and Queen Elizabeth I.

Today the words *prize fight* evoke the image of a boxing match. However, the term developed from the prizes given in professional swordfights in which participants faced injury and even death. British newspaper reports from the 1700s describe fights that were scored by how many wounds each competitor gave and received. During those years, the weapons changed from swords to clubs and staffs, and finally to fists.

The spectacle of violent death continued to draw the public, as revealed by the large numbers of people who gathered to witness public executions. In the United States, as recently as 1934, a crowd of 20,000 gathered for the last execution that allowed unrestricted public participation.

People no longer watch public executions, but they bring violence into their homes through blood-spattered TV shows and videos. They also participate in simulated beatings, shootings, and bloodshedding in ever-more-realistic video games.

For years, researchers have tried to figure out why some people become violent. Everyone deals with conflict day in and day out, yet very few people commit acts of violence. What influences some individuals to respond to conflicts or problems with violence?

Some researchers believe that people are born with a predisposition toward violence. Still others believe the roots of violence lie in a person's upbringing and environment. The answer may be found in a combination or the interaction of these factors. To date, scientists have enjoyed more success in classifying violence than understanding its causes.

COMMON ACTS OF VIOLENCE

As part of a program to provide a uniform annual report of crimes in the United States, the Federal Bureau of Investigation (FBI) has developed general definitions of many forms of violence. Violent crimes include four offenses:

- Homicide consists of murder and nonnegligent manslaughter, defined as the intentional killing of one human being by another. Suicide is not included in this offense. Attempts to murder are classified as aggravated assaults.

- Rape, or forcible rape, defined as sexual intercourse with a female forcibly and against her will. Attempts to commit rape by force or threat of force are also included.

- Robbery, defined as taking or attempting to take anything of value from the care or control of a person by force or threat of force or violence and/or by pulling the victim in fear.

- Assault, or aggravated assault, defined as an unlawful attack by one person upon another for the purpose of inflicting bodily injury, usually involving a weapon. Incidents of displaying or threatening with a gun, knife, or other weapon which could cause bodily harm are included.

Property crimes include the offenses of burglary, larceny/theft, motor vehicle theft, and arson. The offenses involve the taking of money or property, or destroying it. These crimes violate a person's sense of safety and, create fear, but they are not classified as violent by the FBI.

Other forms of violence which may involve law enforcement agencies include simple assault. This occurs when someone attacks, menaces, or intimidates another person without the use of a weapon. Police may also intervene in cases of domestic violence. Also known as family violence, this category includes cases of simple assault that take place in a home environment. Such cases also include spousal or intimate partner abuse, parental or elder abuse, and sibling abuse.

WHAT FACTORS CONTRIBUTE TO VIOLENCE?

National and international agencies increasingly view the problem of violence as a public health issue. The World Health Organization, the global public health body of the United Nations, has issued a report on the worldwide implications of violence. In the United States, the surgeon general, the nation's highest-ranking public health officer, has issued several reports on violence, especially among young people. Agencies like the Centers for Disease Control and Prevention (CDC), the National Institute on Drug Abuse, and the National Institute on Alcohol Abuse and Alcoholism have all worked on violence-related research, as has the Department of Health and Human Services. This research has resulted in identifying a number of symptoms of violence but few cures.

Violence and victims

In 2006, the U.S. Department of Justice estimated that some 6.3 million violent crimes occur in the United States annually and each one had at least one victim.

How do so many people end up as victims of a crime? There are many possible reasons. At times people take risks that put them in danger. For instance, if a person works at night and walks to his or her car alone in the dark, he or she may risk a robbery or an assault. The odds go up considerably if the person is a female. Some people feel a sense of security because nothing has ever happened to them or to anyone they know. Nonetheless, they are still at risk. In many cases, criminals watch their victims for some time before they act.

According to the 2006 National Crime Victimization Survey, 32.8 percent of violent crimes take place between the hours of 6 P.M. and midnight. Another 10.9 percent take place between midnight and 6 A.M. When looking at the location of violent crimes, 20 percent take place at or in the victim's home, while another 12.1 percent take place near the home. A total of 57.5 percent of all violent crimes take place within one mile of a victim's home.

Walking alone at night is only one example of risky behavior. The use of alcohol and drugs also increases one's risk of becoming a victim. Drugs and alcohol can also affect one's judgment on a date. Being intoxicated makes one more vulnerable to rape or robbery. Research shows that people arrested for drug dealing often become involved in this dangerous trade while trying to make enough money to support their own drug habits. Their addiction has forced them into serious and even violent business to pay for it.

These examples serve to reinforce the old saying "Look before you leap." The excitement of the moment may lead people to try things they would not normally do. This happens to everyone at some point in time, and most are lucky enough not to end up in danger because of unwise choices. But the risks are real, and a little planning can save a lot of headaches and heartaches down the road.

On occasion, people find themselves in the wrong place at the wrong time. Large-scale violence usually takes its victims by surprise. Take, for example, the bombing at the Olympic Park during the 1996 Summer Games in Atlanta. Two people were killed in that blast, and another 111 were injured. All count as victims of violence. All were simply in the wrong place at the wrong time. Other examples include the bombing of Oklahoma City's Alfred P. Murrah Federal Building in May 1995 and the destruction of the World Trade Center towers on September 11, 2001. Thousands of innocent victims died in those attacks.

Characteristics of victims

For young people, there is no question that violence is a very real problem. Whatever the type of violent crime, the patterns of victimization indicate that teens are the group hardest hit. According to government statistics, the involvement of young people in violent crimes rises until age 21 and only then begins to fall. According to 2006 data, for every 1,000 teens between the ages of 12 and 15, 46.9 were victims of violent crimes. This jumps to 51.7 for teens between the ages of 16 and 19. In 2007, there were 1,443 teens between the ages of 17 and 19 who were murdered, 88 percent of whom were male.

On average, one of every four high school students has experienced dating violence. Adolescent girls are the more likely victims. Dating violence may involve physical violence, such as striking one's date or forcing sexual activity, but it also includes verbal threats, intimidation, or emotional abuse.

Bullying represents another form of violence often specific to young people. Sometimes the victims accept abuse passively or submissively, sending out the message that they are weak or insecure and that they will probably not fight back if picked on. They may not be weak at all, but their fear sends signals to aggressive schoolmates looking for a target. They might not be as talented or athletic as their peers, or they might be shy and are perceived as weak. Others are called provocative victims. The provocative victim can be anxious or aggressive, generally hot-tempered, and might even pick fights but usually loses them.

When violence occurs in the home between members of the same family, it is called domestic or family violence. Victims of family violence are usually women and children. Men are most often the aggressors in family violence rather than the victims. Victims may not only be physically harmed but also emotionally damaged through constant insults, threats, or humiliation. Women who are victims of family violence often feel as though they cannot leave the relationship because of children, financial security, or fears for their safety.

Hate crimes are acts of violence inflicted on individuals because of their race, ethnicity, gender, or sexual orientation. The most common acts of violence involve hitting, kicking, verbal harassment, or threats. One in seven hate crime victims also has their personal property vandalized with symbols or slogans of an offensive nature.

Violence and perpetrators

Just as no standard description of a victim exists, no standard description of a violent person exists. In 2007, police made approximately 546,161 arrests for violent crimes. Slightly more than 57,000 of those arrested were under the age of 18. Criminal offenders had many different motivations and became violent for a wide variety reasons.

Some scientists theorize that a tendency toward violence may be hereditary, but there is little evidence to support that theory. Most social scientists believe that violence is a learned behavior. People learn how to be violent through what they see in their home and their community. Researchers have spent decades collecting evidence to indicate that young people who watch violence on television are more likely to act in a violent fashion than those who do not. Violent television programs and movies tend to desensitize viewers, who are then less likely to consider the consequences of a violent act or to be shocked by an act of violence.

Psychological studies also support the theory that people who grow up seeing violence perpetrated by adults or who are abused as children are more likely to accept violence as an appropriate means of dealing with conflict as adults.

People who display violent behavior are often deficient in social skills. Rather than using communication to avoid a confrontation or defuse a conflict, they see an act of violence as the first and best solution. Think of the last time a fight happened in your school. Did the people involved make an attempt to discuss the conflict? Did either person clarify what the fight was about? Did anyone try to reach a mutual agreement or find compromise on the issue? Probably not. Fighters see conflict as an opportunity to gain what they want by force, particularly if they are good at fighting. Many schools are now stressing the importance of building conflict resolution skills as a way of discouraging acts of violence.

Social factors also play a role in violent crimes. One of the greatest influences on violent crime is poverty. In areas of the United States where jobs are scarce and neighborhoods are poor, residents may feel that the only way to get what they want in life is to take it. The 2006 National Crime Victimization Survey found that for people in households earning less than $7,500 a year, 63.5 out of 1,000 people become victims of violent crimes, including robbery, murder, rape, and sexual assault. For those from households earning more than $75,000 a year, the victimization rate was only 13.9 per 1,000. Crime is simply more prevalent in poor neighborhoods. Guns are also more prevalent where poverty is high.

Alcohol and other drugs represent another social influence on violence. Simply put, people become less inhibited when they take drugs; they react to situations in ways they would not consider if they were sober. Of all the violent offenders in prison today, more than one-third were committed by individuals under the influence of alcohol or another drug at the time of the crime. In addition, people also commit crimes to *get* the drugs they want. Their addiction is so strong, the psychological and physical need for the drug so great, that they will commit acts of violence to obtain the money to buy drugs.

None of the personal, individual, or social influences mentioned thus far are single reasons someone turns to violence or commits a violent crime. In almost every case, a combination of factors influences a decision to engage in violence.

RISKY BUSINESS SELF TEST: TRUE OR FALSE?

Are you prone to violent behavior? Ask yourself the following questions. Keep a record of your answers on a separate piece of paper.

	Yes, I do	No, I don't
■ Question:		
■ I often engage in arguments with others.	———	———
■ I sometimes engage in arguments with strangers.	———	———
■ I sometimes lose my temper.	———	———
■ I sometimes go to parties where alcohol and weapons are present.	———	———
■ I sometimes go to parties where some partygoers are strangers to everyone else present.	———	———
■ I drink alcohol and hang out with friends.	———	———
■ I carry a weapon in my neighborhood.	———	———
■ I carry a weapon at school.	———	———
■ I belong to a gang.	———	———
■ My behavior is easily influenced by my friends.	———	———
■ I get angry when others do not treat me with respect.	———	———
■ I am easily irritated or annoyed by others.	———	———
■ I make fun of others who are not like me.	———	———
■ I sometimes just need a good argument.	———	———
■ I sometimes daydream about violent activity.	———	———

- I am easily angered while
  I am driving. _____ _____
- I believe my boyfriend/girlfriend
  should do what I tell him/her. _____ _____
- I most enjoy watching shows and
  playing games that have violent
  content. _____ _____
- I will stay in an argument until
  I "win." _____ _____
- I believe that most of the time my
  way of doing things is the right way
  to do things. _____ _____

You may want to ask a person you trust to answer the same questions about your behavior as well. The hardest part of a self-test lies in being honest. Sometimes the way you see yourself is not how others see you. Compare your answers with a friend. If you find that your answers disagree or that you answered more than a few of your questions with "yes," you may want to learn more about violent situations and how they develop.

A-TO-Z ENTRIES

■ ABUSE, CHILD

See: Family Violence

■ ALCOHOL AND VIOLENCE

Alcohol is a mood-altering substance, one of the first used by humans, which can sometimes trigger violent behavior in certain people. Archeologists have found recipes for beer dating back 4,000 years to ancient Egypt and Sumeria. People who consume alcohol can have different reactions. They can become very quiet or very boisterous. In some cases, they become very aggressive.

Scientists and sociologists have studied the relationship between drinking alcohol and becoming violent for decades. They have found that people who use alcohol are much more likely to become violent than those who remain sober. According to the latest data provided by the Bureau of Justice Statistics, in 2002 approximately 1 million violent crimes occurred in which the victim believed that the offender had been drinking. Alcohol played a factor in 66 percent of intimate partner violence. Among spouses who were victims, 75 percent indicated alcohol had been a factor. The 2006 National Crime Victimization Survey indicates that 15.2 percent of all violent crimes involved offenders who had been using alcohol. This number jumps up to 26.8 percent when looking at rapes and sexual assaults.

Alcohol-related violence also has a financial cost. A 2000 report from the Department of Health and Human Services estimated that alcohol abuse cost the United States $184.6 billion in 1998. Those costs included $36.5 billion in lost earnings due to premature death, $9.1 billion for the lost work production of people imprisoned for alcohol-related crimes, and $1 billion in expenses for the victims of those crimes.

How does drinking alcohol encourage violence or make it easier for people to become violent? There is no simple answer. In truth, it may be a chemical change in their brains, a reaction to the environment, or simply what people expect to happen when they pick up a glass.

WHAT ALCOHOL DOES TO YOU

Alcohol is a drug classified as a **depressant**. A depressant is a drug that slows down the reaction time of the central nervous system. It impairs one's ability to react—a major reason why people should not drink and drive. According to the National Highway Traffic Safety

Administration, in 2007 there were 12,998 traffic fatalities in which a driver was found to have a blood alcohol content of .08 or higher.

Fact Or Fiction?

Drinking lets people relax and blow off a little steam. It doesn't really hurt.

The Facts: Some people relax when they drink, but others blow off a little too much steam. According to the American Foundation for Suicide Prevention, alcoholism is a factor in approximately 30 percent of suicides.

In its Campus Dating Violence Fact Sheet, the National Center for the Victims of Crime notes that when the victims knew the offender as a friend, classmate, or intimate partner, 75 percent of the men and 55 percent of the women had been drinking or using drugs before the sexual assault.

Many people incorrectly believe that alcohol is a **stimulant**, a substance that speeds up the central nervous system functions. Young people make this mistake because they feel more free, more open, and more talkative when they drink. Those feelings are a result of a reduction in inhibitions rather than an increase in functioning.

For example, if a young woman is normally shy, she might feel uncomfortable talking to a stranger, even though she might want to do so. Her anxiety tends to keep her from entering a situation that will cause her to be uncomfortable. Under the influence of alcohol, the young woman may be willing to take greater risks. Speaking to someone while under the influence is not a great risk, but she might decide to drive a car.

THEORIES ON THE LINK BETWEEN ALCOHOL AND VIOLENCE

Scientists have yet to establish exactly why violence increases when people drink. However, they have developed several theories on the link between alcohol and violence.

In 1996, scholars from the University of Southern California published a study in the *Psychological Bulletin* analyzing research on the links between alcohol and aggression. One explanation of violent behavior in people who have consumed alcohol is related to reduced inhibition. Consumption of alcohol reduces one's level of inhibition, possibly by reducing the amount of serotonin in the brain. **Serotonin** is a chemical in the brain that scientists believe monitors behavior.

Another theory notes that when people cannot attain a goal, they experience frustration. As the level of frustration increases, so does the level of violence. According to this theory, people who are intoxicated may evaluate situations differently than those who are sober. A problem that they might dismiss as trivial when sober becomes all-important when they are intoxicated. In other words, a person who has been drinking is more likely to overreact than a person who has not been drinking, and is therefore more likely to show aggression.

Q & A

Question: What do I do if I have a friend who drinks and gets violent?

Answer: No one wants to make a friend angry, but situations like this one really determine what kind of friend you are. First, never try to discuss the problem with your friend while he or she is drinking. Alcohol impairs one's ability to think, so there is little chance of a calm discussion.

If your friend begins acting violent, get yourself to a safe place. Wait until the person is sober to discuss the problem. Let the friend know how his or her drinking is affecting your relationship, and that violent behavior may cause greater problems down the road. If you can't discuss the problem with your friend, talk to a trusted adult. Your parent, their parent, or a teacher or school counselor may have good ways to intervene.

ALCOHOL, PERSONALITY, AND VIOLENCE

Some scientists believe there is more to alcohol-related violence than a simple chemical reaction. They add an additional aspect to the relationship—personality. A 2002 article in the journal *Psychology of Addictive Behavior* examined the relationship between those who have an aggressive personality and the likelihood of their becoming violent when drinking. The researchers found that "alcohol-related aggression was strongest among participants who desired an image of power." They also found that when individuals expect alcohol to make them more aggressive, or to show violence, then violence is more likely to occur.

CULTURAL EXPECTATIONS AND ALCOHOL

In much the way that differences in personality result in differences in the way individuals react to alcohol, cultural differences also play a role. A 1998 research paper by the Social Issues Research Centre points out that in some nations—including the United Kingdom, the Scandinavian countries, the United States, and Australia—people expect drinking to result in aggressive and violent behavior. In many Mediterranean countries and parts of South America, people have different cultural assumptions. There, intoxication is expected to result in peaceful behavior.

The report goes on to state that these differences cannot be accounted for by the amount of alcoholic beverages consumed or genetics. They seem to stem from different cultural beliefs about drinking alcohol, its effects, and what is appropriate behavior even while intoxicated.

A 1998 study reported in Marcus Grant and Jorge Litvak's book *Drinking Patterns and Their Consequences* discussed psychological experiments on individuals who believed they were drinking alcoholic beverages but actually were not. Researchers found that people's beliefs about their drinking had more effect on their mood and actions than what they had actually consumed. People who believed that drinking removes inhibitions became more outgoing. Those who believed that drinking puts one in a sexy mood became more amorous. People who believed that drinking results in violence became more aggressive.

Whether alcohol-related violence is a result of chemistry, psychology, sociology, or an interaction among the three, one point remains clear: People lose control when they drink. That loss of control often results in violence, and too often, violence adds to the 105,000 annual deaths attributed to alcohol by the Department of Health and Human Services.

See also: Criminals and Violent Activity; Media and Violence; School Violence; Teens and Violence; Violent Behavior, Causes of

FURTHER READING

Ojeda, Oriana, ed. *Teens at Risk: Opposing Viewpoints*. San Diego: Greenhaven Press, 2003.

Whittington, Dean. *Beaten Into Violence: Anger, Masculinities, Alcohol, Narcotics*. Bloomington, Ind.: AuthorHouse, 2007.

■ ANGER MANAGEMENT

Ability to control anger, often a reaction to stress, in healthy ways. Everyone gets angry at some point in time; it's normal. Anger becomes a problem when a person does not know how to deal with it in a constructive way.

Anger management is necessary when a person cannot control anger that can cause emotional or physical harm to oneself or others. Anger-management programs rely primarily on cognitive behavioral therapies. These therapies help people to change their thinking patterns, which in turn changes negative behavior. Most anger management programs are conducted in group settings, and research indicates that these programs work.

THINKING ERRORS THAT LEAD TO ANGER

Anger management is needed for people who have poor coping skills. If a person does not know healthy ways to handle stress, feelings of frustration and anger will develop. At some point, that anger will lead to aggressive behavior, which may be directed at someone else or at oneself. Typically, instead of making a situation better, people with anger issues make it worse. In turn, this can lead to further anger and frustration.

Anger often becomes a problem for people as a result of faulty thinking patterns. The authors of a 2007 article in the *Journal of Rational-Emotive & Cognitive-Behavioral Therapy* describe the five types of thinking errors related to anger. The first is "misattributing causation." This pattern causes a person to make assumptions about a situation without considering alternative possibilities, that is, to be closed-minded.

The second thinking error is "overgeneralization." This classifying things in the same way, such as, "Everyone is stupid" or "This always happens to me." Instead of viewing people or situations differently, everyone or every occurrence is grouped.

The third error in thinking is "inflammatory labeling." This is when someone views a person or situation in a very negative manner. Using offensive language, such as swearing, is an example of this pattern in a person with anger issues. Even the use of derogatory comments might distort some problem with a person or situation. In other words, using inflammatory remarks can make a person believe that a problem is worse than it actually is.

The fourth thinking error is called "demandingness." This refers to being self-centered—placing your own needs and wants above everyone else's. The last thinking error is "catastrophic evaluations." This, too, is viewing situations as being very negative. However, this error occurs when a person goes a step further than inflammatory labeling and believes he or she does not have the ability or resources to deal with a problem. This not only leads to anger, but the belief that nothing can be done also intensifies the anger.

EFFECTIVENESS OF ANGER-MANAGEMENT PROGRAMS

Most anger-management programs are taught in a group setting. Group therapy sessions are an excellent way for people to better develop social skills and increase their empathy, or perspective-taking, of others. Programs teach people how to use cognitive behavioral techniques to control their anger and behavior. Cognitive behavioral therapy focuses on people changing negative, and often distorted, thinking patterns. As thinking patterns change, so do negative behaviors. Over time, people come to realize how their thinking was problematic and the negative impact it had on their lives. By recognizing this problem, people can then focus on more effective ways to think about problems and react to them in a responsible, rather than an angry, manner.

The authors of a 2006 study in *Behavioural and Cognitive Psychotherapy* examined the effectiveness of an anger-management program for adults using mental-health services. This was a 12-week program that relied on group sessions. Participants had weekly homework assignments designed to help with problem-solving skills and reducing arousal, or agitated states, when confronted with problems. The authors found that the program worked, with participants' gaining better control over their anger. Many participants did drop out of the program, however, and those who dropped out suffered from more depression and self-esteem issues than those who completed the program.

Q & A

Question: Can problems with anger lead to heart disease?

Answer: Yes. There is sufficient evidence to show that anger and other negative emotions can increase the risk of developing heart disease.

A 2009 article in the *Journal of the American College of Cardiology* provided a review of the research on anger and heart disease. The authors found that both anger and hostility increase the risk of heart disease and that anger and hostility had a stronger impact on coronary heart disease in men than in women. Anger not only increased the chances of developing heart disease in healthy people, but it also increased the likelihood of experiencing further problems for those who already have the disease.

An article in a 2007 issue of the *Journal of Child and Adolescent Psychiatric Nursing* provided a review of several anger-management programs. One program was designed for children in grades three to six. The program helped children properly interpret social cues and link these interpretive skills to more appropriate and less aggressive responses. Based on teacher evaluations, those children who went through the program showed improved levels of self-control one year later.

Not all anger-management programs work. The authors reviewed one program for juvenile offenders who were incarcerated, or jailed. The 10-week program was designed to help with social skills, moral reasoning, and anger-control. Although inmates who went through the program showed more signs of pro-social behavior, their ability to better manage anger did not improve.

In a 2008 article in *Family Relations,* the authors focused on an anger-management program for parents. The program, called RETHINK, focused on anger management, parenting skills, child development, and child abuse prevention. RETHINK stands for Recognize, Empathize, Think, Hear, Integrate, Notice, and Keep. It is similar to other cognitive-behavioral programs discussed in this entry. Participants learn about anger, strategies to control it, how to change their thinking habits, and ways to maintain their improved thoughts and actions. In this particular group program, participants met once a week for six weeks. Results of the program were positive, as parents who went through it were better able to control and manage their anger. Family conflict levels decreased, and participants improved their anger-management skills. The authors also discovered that the spouses or partners of the participants also improved their anger-management skills, even though they did not participate in the program.

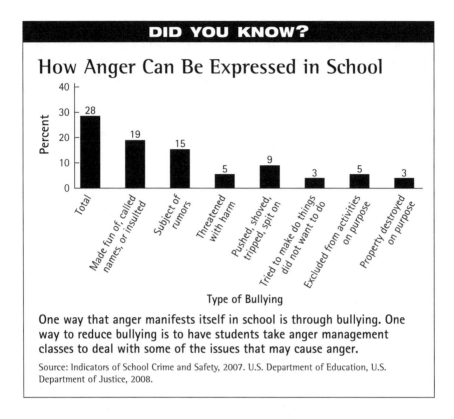

DID YOU KNOW?

How Anger Can Be Expressed in School

One way that anger manifests itself in school is through bullying. One way to reduce bullying is to have students take anger management classes to deal with some of the issues that may cause anger.

Source: Indicators of School Crime and Safety, 2007. U.S. Department of Education, U.S. Department of Justice, 2008.

In 2006, in an article in *Small Group Research,* the authors examined behavioral outcomes at an anger-management therapy course for children with emotional problems. Children from an elementary school participated in this program, which lasted for six sessions. The children learned more about anger, how to tell when they are angry, and basic techniques to control their anger, such as the stop-think-act approach. Results were mixed. Although parents saw changes in their children participating in the program, neither the children nor their teachers noticed any differences.

Q & A

Question: What are some healthy ways to cope with anger?

Answer: Healthy ways to cope with anger involve expressing feelings without causing harm to anyone, including one's self. One of the most common suggestions is to exercise. Whether it is jogging, swimming, lifting weights, or playing sports, exercise is a proven method for reducing anger and stress levels. Another common suggestion for coping with anger is to use relaxation techniques. For example, deep-breathing exercises help calm the body and, at least temporarily, lower anger and stress levels.

PAIN AND ANGER MANAGEMENT

One source of anger is physical pain. Whether it is short-term pain resulting from an injury or constant pain from a **chronic** condition, the presence of pain causes feelings of anger and frustration. This is a problem because when people are angry, their bodies often tense up. Pain can become worse because of anger, which in turn will make a person even angrier. It can be a vicious cycle, and anger-management techniques can help alleviate at least some of the problem.

In *Psychosomatic Medicine,* the authors of a 2006 study examined how anger and anger-management techniques influenced patients with chronic lower back pain. The authors found that patients who suppress their anger and demonstrate a hostile attitude had increased muscle tension in the lower back when they became angry. The authors also discovered that those who suppressed their anger had elevated blood pressure while angry. Also, compared to healthy individuals, people with chronic lower back pain appear to suppress their anger more often and be more hostile in general.

In a 2005 issue of *The Journal of Pain,* the authors of a study examined anger-management styles and their influence on chronic pain in male war veterans. The authors found that veterans with poor anger-coping methods reported higher levels of pain. The authors also found self-efficacy to be important in both anger management and pain experienced. Self-efficacy is the belief a person has in his or her ability to perform an action or behavior. This is related to the concept of "catastrophic evaluations" mentioned earlier. Those people with low self-efficacy, who did not believe they would perform well or at all, had poor anger-management styles and higher levels of pain.

In a 2009 issue of *The British Journal of Psychiatry,* in a particularly interesting study, the authors examined how well cognitive behavioral therapy works in people with **schizophrenia** and who have a history of violence. Treating this patient population can be extremely difficult. The authors found that cognitive behavioral therapy proved to be effective in reducing incidents of aggression during the treatment and the follow-up period. The therapy helped reduce the number of physical incidents of violence as well as reduce the severity of delusions, which are typical of patients with this mental disorder.

Anger-management techniques can work. It is important to consult an adviser or health specialist when investigating which techniques might work best.

See also: Rehabilitation and Treatment of Perpetrators; Road Rage; Violent Behavior, Causes of.

FURTHER READING

Chapman, Gary. *Anger: Handling a Powerful Emotion in a Healthy Way.* Chicago: Northfield Publishing, 2007.

Potter-Efron, Ronald T. *Rage: A Step-by-Step Guide to Overcoming Explosive Anger.* Oakland, Calif.: New Harbinger Publishers, 2007.

■ ASSAULT AND BULLYING

Assault, a legal term for a threat or an attempt to harm another person, and bullying, a kind of assault that is intended to hurt or frighten another person. Bullying may or may not include physical violence. The behavior may consist of a physical attack but may also be limited to verbal bullying (calling a person names, teasing, and taunting him or her) and social bullying (excluding someone from a group or spreading malicious stories about the individual).

An important characteristic of bullying is the inequality of power between the bully and his or her target. The more powerful person or group attacks a less powerful individual.

Consider the following situations: A man knocks a woman down to steal her purse. In an argument over a girlfriend, one man threatens to kill the other, pushing him to the ground. A person tells a coworker, "If you tell the boss I left early, I'll have you fired." Each of these is a case of assault and may be considered a crime. Adults do not accept such behaviors.

Among young people, however, the distinction between an assault and bullying is often blurred. How would the following situations be viewed? A large boy forces other students to give up their lunch money. A new student is knocked down in the school playground because he or she looks "funny." Someone who has broken school rules about smoking threatens witnesses with painful or humiliating abuse if they say anything.

While these incidents are also examples of assault, they are more likely to be called bullying. Some people may even dismiss some of these incidents, saying things like "Boys will be boys," or "Some girls just go through a mean phase."

Since the 1970s, many psychologists have been focusing attention on bullying among young people. According to a report produced by the U.S. Department of Education and the U.S. Department of Justice, in 2005 approximately 28 percent of 12-to-18-year-old students reported that they had been bullied at school. As students progressed through school, they experienced less bullying. For example, about 37 percent of sixth grade students indicated that they had been bullied. This compares to only 20 percent of 12th grade students. Overall, only 9 percent indicated they had been physically bullied (pushed, tripped, shoved, or spit on). However, when physical bullying did occur, 24 percent of students reported that they had been injured. In 2001, a study for the National Institute of Child Health and Human Development found that 29.9 percent of students in the United States were involved in bullying: 13 percent as bullies, 10.6 percent as their targets, and 6.3 percent as both bully and target.

WHAT BULLYING LOOKS LIKE

At any given time, children on a typical schoolyard may be squabbling, teasing, shoving, and even punching one another. How can an observer tell the difference between rough play and bullying? According to experts on bullying, the answer lies in whether a child repeatedly uses violence or threats to influence those around him or her. Experts look for a pattern of behavior.

Bullies also tend to target individuals whom they can continue to bully. They will force their victims to do the things bullies do not want to do or give the bully money. These behaviors generally mark male bullies. When girls bully, they use more indirect, less obvious methods. However, the impact can be just as damaging.

Fact Or Fiction?

All bullies are boys.

The Facts: In 1995, researchers from Canada's York University videotaped children in two Toronto schools. In 52 hours, they recorded 404 bullying incidents, which lasted 37 seconds on average. The majority—72

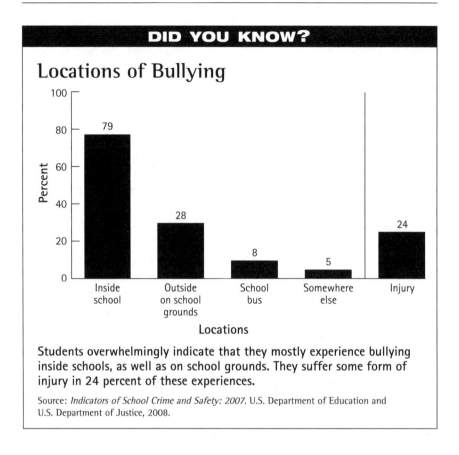

DID YOU KNOW?

Locations of Bullying

Students overwhelmingly indicate that they mostly experience bullying inside schools, as well as on school grounds. They suffer some form of injury in 24 percent of these experiences.

Source: *Indicators of School Crime and Safety: 2007*. U.S. Department of Education and U.S. Department of Justice, 2008.

percent—of the bullies were boys. However, girls were responsible for 28 percent of the bullying.

In her book *Odd Girl Out,* Rachel Simmons, who began her research on female bullying and the psychology of girls at Oxford University, views girls as less likely to punch anyone or knock someone down. Instead, girls use strategies like keeping their target out of the popular group, isolating her, spreading rumors, and damaging her reputation. An observer can often identify a target of female bullying as the girl who sits quietly, almost hiding among the boys, not because she wants to talk to them, but because she has been excluded from the circle of girls.

The female bully will glare at her target across the room, even as she chats with a friend. The impact of such behavior is hurtful to the person on the receiving end. The look says, "You are not wanted here." Feeling unwanted can be very painful, and for some people it can take a lifetime to get over.

THE EFFECTS OF BULLYING

Repeated harassment takes its toll on a bully's victims. According to a 2003 study by Fight Crime: Invest in Kids, a national advocacy group, young people who are bullied are five times more likely to be depressed than other kids. Bullied boys are four times more likely than other boys to be suicidal and bullied girls are eight times more likely than other girls to be suicidal. The report also points out that 75 percent of the attackers in recent cases of school shootings were teens who had been victims of bullying.

Bullying also has consequences for the perpetrators, the individuals who bully. In his book *Understanding and Managing Bullying,* Delwyn Tattum cites a 22-year study which found that boys described by their peers as very aggressive (displaying bullying behavior) had a one in four chance of becoming criminals by the age of 30, compared to a one in 20 chance among other male students. The study also found that as these boys grew older, they acted aggressively towards their wives and children and tended to have children who behaved aggressively.

TEENS SPEAK

Mean Girls

Janet is a 21-year-old college junior. She was bullied by a group of girls all through high school.

"I was hated in school. I had bright red hair, was very skinny, and wore glasses. Nothing about me fit in with the 'in' crowd." Janet doesn't look up, keeping her eyes on her clasped hands. "And they let me know it. The girl who used to be my best friend quit talking to me because the cheerleading captain said it would not look good to be seen with a loser."

Her hands are tightly clenched together. "It turned out that a boy I really liked asked me out only because someone told him I'd do 'anything' to have him like me. When I wouldn't do 'anything,' he was gone. I spent most of my time alone because I was afraid of what people had said about me. By the time I was a senior, I just wanted to graduate and get away from there, because I thought it would be over. But it wasn't."

Janet's fingers are so tight, they've gone white. "I didn't see those girls after high school, but I felt so badly about myself that I couldn't get my life to work. At one point I even thought about ending it all, you know, committing suicide, but I couldn't do it. It took almost a year of counseling before I realized that I had some value, but it will take several more before I am over it, and I will never forget it."

DEALING WITH BULLYING

Are you a bully? To answer that question, take a hard look at yourself. Try to determine if you do things, say things, arrange things in such a way as to control others. People who bully make decisions about others based on what others have told them instead of what they know. Find out what others are like, and learn to accept that not all people will view the world the same way you do. That knowledge is part of becoming mature.

Perhaps you are not a bully but you support others who bully. You may occasionally be around when a friend or classmate is threatening others or spreading rumors. You have choices. You can ignore the behavior or suggest a different, more positive way to work out differences. Many people complain about peer pressure, the pressure or need to go along with others in a group. Making your disapproval plain is an opportunity to use peer pressure in a positive way.

Finally, learn how to resolve conflicts peacefully. It is a skill that can be learned in much the way you learn to shoot a basketball or sing. Like other skills, it also takes practice. Not only will it help you, but your friends will notice as well. It can be your chance to help create a better school for everyone. Things do not, and will not, change overnight and there will be those people who you simply cannot reach. Even so, at least you'll be making an effort to improve your corner of the world.

See also: Criminals and Violent Activity; Media and Violence; School Violence; Teens and Violence; Violent Behavior, Causes of

FURTHER READING

Carter, Jay, and Kathy Noll. *Taking the Bully by the Horns.* Pennsylvania: Unicorn Press, 1998.

Haber, Joel, and Jenna Glatzer. *Bullyproof Your Child for Life: Protect Your Child from Teasing, Taunting, and Bullying for Good.* New York: Perigee Trade, 2007.

■ COMMUNITIES AND VIOLENCE

Communities are groups of people who live in a particular local area, often bound together by economic, political, and social ties. How does violence affect communities? The World Health Organization (WHO), the global health authority of the United Nations, issued the *World Report on Violence and Health* in 2002. This study reported:

- 1.6 million deaths from violence
- 520,000 homicides
- 815,000 suicides
- 310,000 war-related deaths

North and South America, including the United States, had the second-highest homicide rate in the world. Like it or not, violence affects everyone. In many ways, individuals are products of their physical and social environments. A person's outlook and expectations are shaped by their home life and their neighborhood. The more violence a person lives with, the more profound are its effects.

A 1995 article in the *American Psychologist* discusses a situation called **chronic community violence** (CCV). Places marked by CCV have frequent and continuous exposure to the use of guns, knives, drugs, and random violence. Many of these places are poor, urban neighborhoods that have been compared to war zones. Like people trapped in a war zone, residents not only face the threat of physical harm, but also psychological danger.

Fact Or Fiction?

Crime is not just a problem in the inner city.

The Facts: A 2004 report from the U.S. Department of Justice on school crime and safety found that 12- to 18-year-old students in urban areas were at greater danger of facing serious violent crime. For crimes like theft, however, the study found suburban students had a greater risk than urban students while in school, while students in rural areas had the same crime risk as urban students outside of school. Like it or not, crime—even violent crime—is everywhere.

COMMUNITIES THAT NEGLECT
REPORTS OF VIOLENCE

According to the article in the *American Psychologist,* in areas where CCV is widespread, unchecked violence has a significant impact on those who live there. Children in such environments grow up believing that violence is a part of everyday life. Young children often cling to parents and caregivers, and may be fearful of exploring the world outside their homes. As they grow older, their early experiences with violence may encourage aggressive behavior. These young people may be more likely to respond to frustration with violence than young people in safer environments. Young people who grew up in violent surroundings may also have a nagging feeling that they do not "fit in" anywhere.

A 2003 study of youths in Los Angeles for the *Journal of Education* found that over 50 percent of the children in the neighborhood surveyed had been hit, slapped, or punched. Over 40 percent had been chased, threatened, or had hard objects thrown at them. More than 25 percent had experienced violence as a way of persuading them to do something they did not want to do. The researchers found that these children did not perform well academically. The more violence they had been exposed to, the lower their scores in school. Many suffered from depression and had low energy and even lower expectations of performing well in school.

A 2008 study in *Psychiatria* found that experiencing physical violence during childhood has emotional consequences. The authors discovered that children who had been victims of violence experienced anxiety, anger, and reported feeling a lack of control. Further, these children were at an increased risk for harming themselves and attempting to commit suicide.

COMMUNITY VIOLENCE-PREVENTION STRATEGIES

Overcoming the negative influence of violence requires action from the entire community. The World Health Organization suggests several measures to increase safety and reduce violence at the community level, including:

- Utilizing public education to target communities or community entities like schools and businesses
- Modifying the physical environment by creating better lighting and safe routes to walk
- Ensuring the existence of after-school programs for youths
- Preparing police, health professionals, and educators to address violence with special training
- Developing community policing groups
- Coordinating efforts for a unified approach to dealing with violence

Using these strategies and others, cities across the United States have managed to reduce crime—and violence—in recent years.

WHAT CAN BE DONE

Some of these efforts are already under way in many communities, many of which have experienced success. Organizing a community to address violence means bringing many groups together. The 1997 guide *Building Coalitions 101,* issued by the advocacy group known as the Community Anti-Drug Coalition of America, offers a seven-step program to identify problems and to recruit help from parents and local service organizations. According to the 2008 Coalition annual report, people in more than 5,000 communities are successfully working to reduce drug use and violence.

An example of creating coalitions from the national to the local level was the partnership between the American Psychological Association (APA) and MTV (Music Television) in the late 1990s to help prevent school violence. After a series of shootings at schools, the two organizations developed a program called Warning Signs. The effort was launched with the broadcast of a special documentary on MTV which featured a toll-free number that young people could call to request more information. The U.S. Secretary of Education helped promote the program to 60,000 educators, and APA members across the country joined in, offering community outreach. Psychologists in numerous cities and towns conducted youth forums and worked with church groups, boys and girls clubs, and other youth organizations. Special kits helped these volunteers prepare presentations and work with community leaders both to create grassroots activities and promote them.

Most efforts to address local issues are much smaller in scale, but the processes that enable their success are similar. Many communities also have support systems established to help individuals. Self-help groups are commonly found throughout the nation, with support in dealing with such issues as alcoholism and drug abuse, both of which can lead to violence. A look in the local phone book may reveal help lines for those who are coping with child abuse, sex crimes, or family violence.

For those having difficulty changing violent behaviors on their own, personal counseling is an option. Trained professionals can work with perpetrators of violence to assist in learning appropriate nonviolent methods of expressing feelings and opinions. Local health departments often offer counseling or programs to help those who wish to control violent behavior. Violence is a community issue, and it will take a community effort to make neighborhoods safe.

Q & A

Question: How can I reduce violence in my community?

Answer: Many people feel overwhelmed by the problem of violence. What can a single person do? Community action is about uniting the work of many individuals.

The National Youth Violence Prevention Resource Center suggests many ways in which young people can become involved in community-based action against violence. You could volunteer with existing organizations in your town or city. Check and see if your school or a community group already has programs to prevent or counter violence. Another opportunity is to work with local government, serving on planning boards.

If there are no existing organizations in your area, you may follow the lead of many young people by stepping into the gap and creating your own.

The Centers for Disease Control offers information on the Best Practices of Youth Violence Prevention. The information can be found online at: http://www.cdc.gov/ncipc/dvp/bestpractices.htm.

The CDC also maintains a separate Web site that focuses on violence prevention strategies and information. That Web site is: http://www.safeyouth.org.

See also: Drugs and Violence; Gang Violence; Social Costs of Violence

FURTHER READING

Anderson, Elijah. *Code of the Street: Decency, Violence, and the Moral Life of the Inner City.* New York: W. W. Norton, 2000.

Thorton, Timothy N., Carole A. Craf, Linda L. Dahlberg, Barbara S. Lynch, and Katie Baer. *Youth Violence Prevention: A Sourcebook for Community Action.* Hauppauge, N.Y.: Novinka Books, 2007.

■ CONFLICT RESOLUTION

See: School Violence

■ CRIMINALS AND VIOLENT ACTIVITY

People who habitually break the law, often committing the crime of theft. While some forms of crime such as fraud do not require violence, for most criminals, violent behavior is part of the job.

LEGAL DEFINITIONS

The Federal Bureau of Investigation (FBI) maintains the Uniform Crime Reporting Program, an effort to generate nationwide crime statistics. In this annual report, the FBI divides violent crimes into four categories:

- **Murder and nonnegligent manslaughter:** the willful (nonnegligent) killing of one human being by another
- **Aggravated assault:** an unlawful attack by one person upon another for the purpose of inflicting severe or aggravated bodily injury. This type of assault is usually

accompanied by the use of a weapon or other means likely to produce death or cause bodily harm. Attempts involving the display or threat of a gun, knife, or other weapon are included because serious personal injury is likely to occur if the assault is completed.

- **Forcible rape:** forcing a person to submit to sexual intercourse against his or her will. Assaults or attempts to commit rape by force or the threat of force are also included. The category does not include statutory rape (a sexual act between an adult and a minor; by law no minor can consent to sex with an adult).

- **Robbery:** taking or attempting to take something of value by force or by threat of violence

LAWS

Laws are the rules that govern a community. Criminal laws usually ban specific acts considered harmful to individuals and the community as a whole. These laws often specify punishments for offenders. Violent offenses usually fall into one of two classifications. **Misdemeanors** are lesser crimes. Offenses include theft of items of little value, disturbing the peace, simple assault and battery, drunk driving without injury to others, and public intoxication. Those convicted of a misdemeanor usually pay a fine or spend up to a year in jail. **Felonies** are more serious crimes, punishable by a term in a state or federal prison, with a minimum sentence of one year, and, in some cases, the death penalty.

The number of laws, lawbreakers, and court cases in the United States is staggering. In the last 20 years, concern over the operation of the courts has led to new laws setting guidelines for the administration of the legal system.

In 2007, the Bureau of Justice Statistics released a report stating that violent offenders, on average, completed 66 percent of their sentences, or 56 months out of an average 85-month sentence. Because of community demand for jail time for those convicted of violent crimes, many states began adopting **truth-in-sentencing laws.** These laws require that violent offenders finish at least 85 percent of their sentence. In the 1994 Crime Act, the federal government promised money for more prisons to states enacting this type of law. If criminals were going to be staying in prison longer, the state would need more room to house them. The first state to adopt a truth-in-sentencing law was Washington in 1984. Since that time, over half of the states have passed laws that mandate a minimum percentage of time to be served by persons convicted of violent crimes.

In response to the increase in violent offenses and drug-related crimes in the 1980s, and to address differences in how individual judges sentenced criminals for the same crimes, the federal government created **mandatory sentencing laws.** These laws provide judges in federal courts with guidelines for sentencing based on the seriousness of the crime, previous convictions for the crime, and whether the accused has been cooperative with the courts.

Concern over repeat offenders of serious crimes led to the "three strikes, and you're out" laws. These state statutes establish tougher sentencing for criminals who repeatedly commit felonies. In most cases, if the accused has been convicted of a third offense, he or she faces 25 years to life in prison without the opportunity for parole. Washington State passed the first of these laws in 1993. In 1994, California voters approved a similar measure. At present, 24 states have laws that aim at keeping repeat offenders in prison. Variations exist from state to state as to what types of crimes qualify for this sentencing. For example,

DID YOU KNOW?

Estimated Average Time to Be Served Under Truth-in-Sentencing Laws

Most serious offense	New Sentencing Maximum sentence (years)	Minimum sentence (years)	Estimated Time to Be Served 85% of sentence	75% of sentence	50% of sentence
Violent offenses	104	73	88	78	52
Murder	253	214	215	190	127
Rape	140	72	119	105	70
Robbery	101	60	86	76	51
Assault	72	45	61	54	36

Note: Excludes life, death, and without-parole sentencing

Source: Truth-in-Sentencing in State Prisons, Bureau of Justice Statistics, 1999.

in some states, all three felonies must be violent offenses. Other states require that the first two offenses be violent, while the third can be any felony. A federal "three strikes" law also exists for those convicted of federal offenses.

LAW ENFORCEMENT

The job of investigating crimes and apprehending the perpetrators falls on officers of various jurisdictions. According to the Bureau of Justice Statistics, in 2004, there were approximately 446,794 police officers. In the nation, at both state and local levels, there were approximately 731,903 police officers. At the federal level, an additional 104,884 people were authorized to make arrests, representing dozens of different government agencies, including the FBI, Secret Service, Immigration and Naturalization Service, U.S. Customs Service, and Federal Bureau of Prisons.

In many towns of moderate size, a police department consists of a police chief, several officers, and various other professionals who have investigative or administrative duties. The amount of protection a local force can provide has a direct effect on the amount of violence in the community. The greater the protection, the less violence there was in the community. A 1996 study in the journal *Criminology* found that each additional police officer on duty in a city results in approximately 24 fewer crimes.

PUNISHMENT

After a lawbreaker is convicted in court, he or she is sentenced. Depending on the seriousness of the crime, and whether the case is in a county, state, or federal court, the judge will determine the appropriate sentence for the crime. In county court, the judge has considerable flexibility in determining what the sentence will be. One option is jail. If the crime is serious enough, a lawbreaker can typically be sentenced up to one year in county jail. Usually, if the crime is more serious, the case is tried in state or federal court, where a year's prison time is usually the minimum sentence.

Another sentencing option is **probation**—in which a convicted defendant is released under supervision as long as certain conditions are met. Probation has the requirement that if the person convicted of the crime gets into any additional trouble, the full sentence is enforced.

A third option is to have the lawbreaker pay a fine. The amount of the fine depends on the crime and usually includes an additional fee called court costs—the costs associated with the trial. Yet another sentencing option might be community service. Many judges will decide that rather than send a person to jail they will have him or her help make the community a better place. Some people who perform community service do menial jobs, such as picking up trash along the highways. More often, such service involves an assignment to work with a group of people connected to the crime. For example, a person arrested for drunk driving may be required to perform 100 hours of community service talking to youngsters about the dangers of drinking and driving, and the consequences they will face if they are caught.

When children and teens get in trouble with the law, they are tried in juvenile courts, state courts set aside for young people under the age of 18. (A few states, however, define juveniles as young people who are under the age of 16 or 17.) The goal of juvenile courts is to help young people in trouble rather than treat them as hardened criminals. Illinois established the first juvenile court in 1899.

In juvenile court, those found guilty of a crime are called delinquents. They are often released into the custody of parents or guardians and required to undergo counseling or do community service. When sentences are imposed, they are short, lasting only as long as the offender remains a juvenile. These sentences are usually served in juvenile facilities that emphasize rehabilitation. Juvenile records may also be sealed to protect the privacy of the young offenders.

Between 1985 and 1994, an increase in youth violence alarmed people nationwide, and many demanded changes in the juvenile justice system. Many states passed laws required that young people be tried as adults for serious offenses such as murder.

Crime often involves violence. Violent crimes influence laws, which in turn can seriously affect the lives of people, especially young people, who become caught up in the legal system.

See also: Drugs and Violence; Gang Violence; Homicide; Legal Interventions; Rehabilitation and Treatment of Perpetrators; Weapons of Violence

FURTHER READING

Dudley, William, ed. *Crime and Criminals: Opposing Viewpoints.* San Diego: Greenhaven Press, 1989.

Hawkins, Darnell F. *Violent Crime: Assessing Race and Ethnic Differences.* New York: Cambridge University Press, 2003.

■ DATING VIOLENCE
See: Teens and Violence

■ DOMESTIC VIOLENCE
See: Family Violence

■ DRUGS AND VIOLENCE
Substances taken into the body to treat a disease, affect one's mental processes, satisfy a dependence, or attempt suicide. The drugs most associated with violence, however, are illegal substances taken for their effect on one's mental processes.

According to the 2007 Monitoring the Future survey, 21.9 percent of 12th grade students admitted trying an illegal drug within the previous 30 days. This compares to 19.3 percent of college students and 18.9 percent of young adults. When examining specific drug use, 18.8 percent of high school seniors admitted to smoking marijuana in the previous 30 days. Two percent admitted to using cocaine, 1.6 percent admitted to using ecstasy, and 3.7 percent admitted to using amphetamines. These figures decrease for older age groups (college students and young adults).

A 1985 article in the *Journal of Drug Issues* set forth a three-point connection between drugs and violence, which was accepted by the National Institute of Justice (NIJ) as a basic concept in antidrug policies. This concept was subsequently used by the NIJ and the government to explain why drugs are dangerous. First, violence occurs because of the physical effects of drugs. Second is the economic compulsion—drug users often resort to crime to pay for drugs. Finally, the article identified systemic violence—essentially the cost of doing business in an illegal market. Disputes between drug dealers are often settled with guns, and the vast amount of unlawful cash draws robbers. Along with conflicts over price, selling of fake drugs, and run-ins with the law, the world of drugs is a violent place both for sellers and buyers.

Q & A

Question: Why does drug use seem to get out of control so fast?

Answer: One reason is tolerance—a physical reaction after being introduced to a drug. A user's system becomes accustomed to having the drug present and requires a larger dose to attain the effect of pleasure, or even to feel normal.

However, the more an addict uses a drug, the more the body needs. Eventually, the user is totally focused on attaining the drug, and any fun associated with drug taking disappears. Even with less addictive drugs, the users tend to become focused on thoughts and plans for the next time they will be getting high. At that point, users do not control the drug; the drug controls the users.

TYPES OF DRUGS

Illicit drugs fall into six groups. **Depressants** like chloral hydrate and pentobarbital slow the functioning of the nervous system. **Sedatives** like Valium and Xanax reduce anxiety in the user. **Stimulants** speed up the nervous system, raising heart rate and blood pressure. Cocaine, **crack**, and **Benzedrine** are all examples of stimulants.

Narcotics like codeine and morphine serve as painkillers in the medical field, but illegal drugs such as opium and **heroin** also belong to this group. **Cannabis** is another name for marijuana. Many teens consider marijuana to be harmless. Only 34.5 percent of young people considered monthly marijuana use to be highly risky, according to the government's 2007 National Survey of Drug Use and Health. In comparison, 68.8 percent of the respondents considered a pack-a-day cigarette habit to be highly risky. However, according to the American College of Emergency Physicians, cannabis distorts the senses, causes memory loss, damages the immune system, and, in some cases, creates hallucinations and fills users with paranoid fears. It also produces many of the same smoking hazards as cigarettes.

Hallucinogens, like LSD, PCP, and mescaline, distort reality, so that users see and hear things that are not really there. The effects of hallucinogens can last for hours, but the potential for flashbacks (reliving the experience at a later date without taking the drug) can last for years. The last group is **inhalants**. Anything sniffed is included in this group. Spray paint, glue, gas and cleaning products are common inhalants. Users feel dizzy and lightheaded. Inhalants may also stop heartbeat and respiration.

In a 2001 report, the Office of National Drug Control Policy estimated that in 2000, Americans spent $36 billion for cocaine, $11 billion on marijuana, $10 billion on heroin, $5.4 billion on metamphetamine, and $2.4 billion on other drugs. Totaling those figures offers nearly 65 billion reasons for violence in a hugely profitable criminal enterprise.

Fact Or Fiction?

Most kids try smoking pot in high school, so it's not a big deal.

The Facts: Answering the 2007 Monitoring the Future survey, 41.8 percent of students in grade 12 said that they had tried marijuana once or more. Nearly 60 percent *do not* smoke marijuana.

Smoking pot is a big deal. In 2003, the magazine *New Scientist* reported a study of twins. One of the pair began using marijuana before the age of 17, while the other didn't. The early users were two to five times more likely to use harder drugs or become dependent on alcohol than their nonusing twin. A 1994 study by Columbia University's Center on Addiction and Substance Abuse found that young people who used marijuana were 17 times more likely to use cocaine than young people who did not smoke pot.

INTRAVENOUS DRUG USE

Intravenous means inside or into a vein. One of the fastest ways to introduce drugs into the body is by way of the bloodstream. Drug addicts inject many substances, including narcotics such as morphine, Demerol, Percodan, Percocet, and dilaudid. The most common drug abused by intravenous injection is heroin. Several music stars have died from either intentional or unintentional drug overdoses. Recent examples include Michael Jackson, DJ AM (Adam Goldstein), and Jonathan Melvoin (Smashing Pumpkins). Although these musicians were celebrated because of their music, their legacy will include the manner in which they died.

Intravenous drug use is a very dangerous practice. Users expose themselves to the risks of disease transmission and **overdose.** Injected drugs like heroin can cause users to become highly agitated if their "high" is disturbed. The narcotic effect of the drug makes concentration difficult, leaving users easily startled. The way heroin affects the brain intensifies feelings of fear and suspicion, possibly triggering angry or violent outbursts.

Self-violence is also a real possibility. When a drug begins to wear off, the user may experience depression—a feeling of intense sadness and hopelessness. Such emotions have been known to lead to suicide.

TEENS SPEAK

Not a Good Buzz

Sean is a high school student who hopes to make up the class work for junior year—depending on the decision of his town's juvenile court.

"I thought I could handle it. We all did. It started in the ninth grade, smoking a little weed between classes in our friend's car. After a while though, that got boring, so we upped the ante."

He shakes his head. "The first time Freddie brought crack to school, we all looked at him like he was totally nuts. Smoking dope was one thing, but crack? No way. In the end, though, we did it."

Sean's lips twist as if he is tasting something nasty. "I was the last one. The guys were dogging me so much, I tried it just to make them shut up. It was the best high I'd ever had. So good, that I wanted to do it all the time. I thought I was in control, but the drug had me. We were all about finding the money to get some more rock."

He jams his hands into the pockets of his prison cover-all. "We went to the next town over to hit the convenience store. Freddie held the gun while I grabbed the cash. I was already headed out the door when I heard the shot.

"So here I sit in Juvie, waiting on my trial. I just keep thinking, 'We were just getting a buzz, having some fun.' But it doesn't look that way now."

DRUGS AND LOSS OF CONTROL

When a drug user starts out, everything seems good–very good. For a small dose, often given free or for a low price, many users experience tremendous pleasure.

Even at that early stage, however, dangers exist. Drugs can impair the user's thought processes, leading to violence. The substances that commonly cause such reactions are stimulants like cocaine, alcohol, and hallucinogens like PCP. Another class of drugs that may cause physiological violence is steroids. Many young people, especially males, turn to these substances to build up muscle mass. However, a side effect of the drug is violent outbursts known as **steroid or 'roid rage.**

As time goes on, repeated doses of a drug lead to **addiction.** The user's body and mind are in constant need of the drug—not to feel pleasure, but to feel normal. **Tolerance,** the process by which the body needs larger and larger doses of a drug, sets in. The heavier the dose, the greater the cost an addict must pay.

If a user cannot get the drug, he or she may suffer from **withdrawal** as the body responds to the absence of what has become a necessary element. Symptoms range from restlessness and irritability to, in the case of heroin, life-threatening reactions. A person in pain and on edge can react unpredictably. As symptoms become more painful, an addict will do anything, including committing a crime, to raise the money for the next fix.

Research has repeatedly shown a relationship between drug use and engaging in criminal behavior. The authors of a 2008 study in the journal *Aggression and Violent Behavior* found such a relationship exists. Drug users were almost three to four times more likely than nondrug users to engage in criminal behavior. Drug users were, on average, six times more likely to engage in shoplifting and almost three times as likely to engage in prostitution. Further, drug users were two and a half times more likely to commit burglaries and almost twice as likely to commit robberies.

A 2009 study in the journal *European Addiction Research* produced similar findings. Overall, those who used drugs were twice as likely to engage in violence when compared to those who did not use drugs.

Addiction means that users *must* buy drugs, and they must buy them from criminals, because the drugs are illegal. Law enforcement agencies target drug dealers, who are also targeted by business rivals. As an illegal cash business, drug sellers also attract other criminals hoping to get rich quickly. Unable to control their need for drugs, addicts deal with drug dealers. Like it or not, in doing so, the users put themselves in the cross fire of the violence that swirls around the drug business.

Drugs impair the judgment and sometimes create violent physical reactions. The need for drugs often drives users to crime. At the same time, the very act of buying drugs can put addicts in danger. However pleasurable, exciting, and glamorous the world of drugs may seem, its reality is very violent—and often deadly.

See also: Criminals and Violent Activity; Gang Violence; Social Costs of Violence

FURTHER READING

Avraham, Regina. *The Downside of Drugs*. New York: Chelsea House Publishers, 1988.

Ford, Jean Otto. *Rural Crime and Poverty: Violence, Drugs, and Other Issues*. Broomall, Pa.: Mason Crest Publishers, 2007.

■ FAMILY VIOLENCE

Violent activities that take place among members of a family. Because the violence usually takes place in the home, family violence is also called **domestic violence**. Family violence is a hard thing to talk about. Children do not want to admit that their mothers or fathers hit them, or that mother and father hit each other. It is hard enough to survive physical mistreatment. Adding social embarrassment to the violence is something most young people would prefer to avoid. But the fact is, family violence is a real problem that occurs regardless of whether a family is rich or poor, urban and rural, or a one-parent or two-parent household.

Fact Or Fiction?

When adults warn children about abuse, they should only warn them about strangers.

The Facts: According to the organization RAINN (Rape, Abuse & Incest National Network), research shows that approximately 73 percent of all sexual assaults are committed by someone whom the victim knows.

In its pamphlet *Child Protection,* the National Center on Missing and Exploited Children urges that parents train their children to watch out for certain types of behavior rather than certain types of people. To a child, a stranger is someone who looks unusual or odd. Therefore, a child might talk to someone he or she does not know if that person looks "normal" or average.

CHILD ABUSE

The U.S. Department of Health and Human Services (HHS) keeps track of child abuse on a national level. According to HHS statistics, nearly 1 million youngsters were abused or neglected in 2001. That number means for every 500 students in your school and others like it, six or seven children were probably abused last year. It happens to children of all ages, of all nationalities, and to both boys and girls. Generally, abuse of children involves **physical abuse, sexual abuse, emotional abuse,** or **neglect.**

The Committee on the Training Needs of Health Professionals to Respond to Family Violence has developed a number of definitions regarding abuse. Physical abuse is inflicting physical harm by punching, beating, kicking, biting, burning, shaking, or other actions that result in damage.

Sexual abuse is forcing children or adults who are unable to comprehend and/or give consent to engage in sexual activities. This abuse includes all forms of incest, rape, fondling genitals, and commercial exploitation through prostitution or the production of pornographic materials. Neglect is the failure of a loved one or caregiver to provide basic physical, emotional, medical, or educational needs.

The American Medical Association defines emotional abuse as threatening, humiliating, ignoring, or other emotional mistreatment of a child. This type of abuse includes the corruption of a child—for example, when adults introduce children to antisocial activities like crime, sexual activity or pornography, and drug or alcohol use.

A 2001 report from the National Child Abuse and Data System (NCANDS) revealed that parents were the most likely people to abuse children—they are responsible in 80.9 percent of abuse cases. According to 2002 statistics from the Administration for Children and Families, part of the HHS, more than 1,300 children die from abuse each year. Of the children killed, 76 percent were under the age of four.

Q & A

Question: If I am experiencing violence at home, who can I call for help?

Answer: If there is an adult in your life that you can trust, start there. If not, many organizations can help. A good place to start is by calling ChildHelp USA at 1-800-4ACHILD (1-800-422-4453). Your call will be kept confidential, and you can remain anonymous if you want. The group has people on the phones trained to give advice and to help you move forward with your life.

DISCIPLINE VERSUS ABUSE

Dictionary definitions of **discipline** range from "training to improve strength or self-control" to "punishment." Parents have long debated whether physical discipline, primarily spanking, is abusive. Some disapprove of any form of physical aggression toward a child. Others believe physical discipline such as spanking can be an effective way to get children to change their behavior.

According to the American Academy of Pediatrics (AAP), more than 90 percent of American families use spanking, which is defined as the use of an open hand "to a child's buttocks without causing injury, and with the intent to modify behavior of the child." In its policy statement, however, the AAP regards spanking as an ineffective strategy, with a potential for abuse. A 2002 article in *Psychological Bulletin* reports that two-thirds of incidents of parent-child abuse start out as an attempt at discipline.

Child neglect as a form of abuse

According to a 2008 report by the U.S. Department Health and Human Services, 64.2 percent of child abuse cases involve neglect. Neglect occurs when a parent or caregiver—like a grandparent or child-care provider—fails to meet the child's needs. The neglect may be visible, such as when a child is not fed on a regular basis and seems noticeably thinner than his or her peers, when he or she appears at school in torn clothing or missing pieces of clothing such as socks or shoes, or when the child's home is unsafe to live in.

Other forms of neglect may not be as visible. On religious grounds or due to other beliefs, some parents withhold medical care from a child. Other parents may believe that working and supporting the family takes priority over schooling, so the child may be removed from school at an early age. Today education is considered a basic need for all children. According to the 2008 report, 776,758 reports of child maltreatment were substantiated.

Intimate partner abuse

An intimate partner is an individual with whom an adult has a sexual relationship. The individual may be a current or former spouse, a live-in boyfriend or girlfriend, or a dating companion. Whenever these relationships result in physical, sexual, or emotional violence, they are considered instances of **intimate partner abuse.**

Women are the victims of intimate partner violence far more often than men. Department of Justice statistics for 2000 report that 20 percent of violent acts against women are committed by intimate partners. The 1998 National Violence Against Women Survey (NVAWS) conducted by the National Institute of Justice and the Centers for

Disease Control and Prevention found that 24.8 percent of all women have experienced this form of violence at some point in their life. Men report similar violence, but in lesser numbers. In the NVAWS study, only 7.6 percent of men said they have experienced intimate partner abuse at some point in their lives.

In 2001, the University of California at Berkeley prepared training materials for professionals in the Child Welfare Service. These included lists of risk factors for domestic violence and severe violence. Among the risk factors are poor communication skills, quickness to irritation, and a rigid belief in traditional sex roles (a "macho" attitude).

Another major factor in marital violence is alcohol abuse. According to the University of California, about 60 percent of batterers abuse alcohol. Drinking impairs a person's ability to make sound decisions. In a troubled relationship marked by conflict, alcohol can lead to greater aggression and violence. A 2003 study in the *Journal of Consulting and Clinical Psychology* reported that on days when men engaged in heavy drinking, they were almost 20 times more likely to become violent than on days when they did not drink.

TEENS SPEAK

It's Hard to Be a Survivor . . .
But What Choice Do I Have?

Jenna is a 19-year-old single mother. She's taking remedial classes and hopes to attend college.

"When I was six years old, the man my mother was living with began molesting me. I remember waking up one night to find him rubbing me all over, this stupid grin on his face. He kept coming to my room until I was 11. When my mother started to realize something wasn't right, she began sleeping in my room with me. But it was way too late; the damage was done."

Jenna shakes her head. "As I got older, Mom thought I was being rebellious. I just thought that smoking and drinking with my friends after school was better than going home. I met a boy my senior year in high school—I thought he was pretty cool. We would listen to music together or have a smoke. One day he invited me to his house to hang out. We were just listening to music and talking and the next thing I knew he was lying on top of me."

Her voice gets very low. "I didn't want sex, I didn't want to be touched. But I froze. Everything from the time I was very young rushed through my head, and I froze. I couldn't fight, or speak . . . I just lay there. When he was done, he told me not to be such a tease and to just relax. Less than a month later, I knew I was pregnant, but he was long gone."

Jenna takes a deep breath. "Now I'm trying to raise my little baby, and I've decided to talk about what happened. I see a counselor a couple times each month, and I am trying to make sense of it all—not that it's easy. There are good days and bad, but I owe it to myself, and now my child, to get my life on track."

ELDER ABUSE

Elder abuse is abusive acts against older persons—usually people over the age of 60. Social scientists only began studying this form of abuse in the 1970s. They now recognize that elder abuse includes many different types of abuse, including those associated with child and spousal abuse (physical, emotional, sexual, neglect). However, elder abuse can also include financial exploitation, abandonment, and self-neglect. The American Psychological Association's Web site on elder abuse points out that in studies from 1994 to 2004, reported cases of elder abuse have consistently risen, from 117,000 to 241,000. A 2006 report by The National Center on Elder Abuse estimates that 191,908 reports of elder abuse were substantiated in 2004. Another 46,794 reports of self-neglect were substantiated for the same year.

CYCLES OF VIOLENCE

Attitudes about violence are established in childhood. The surgeon general, the nation's chief public health officer, issued a report on youth violence in 2001 that commented in part on 40 years of research and discussion on the impact that watching violence on television has on children. How much worse are the effects of seeing violence on a daily basis in real life? Children growing up in violent homes see their mother humiliated, battered, or sexually abused. They stand a chance of being beaten themselves.

DID YOU KNOW?

Persons Raped or Physically Assaulted in Their Lifetime, by Gender of Victim

Type of Assault	Percentage[a]		Numbers[b]	
	Women	Men	Women	Men
	(n= 8,000)	(n= 8,000)	(100,697,000)	(92,748,000)
Total rape	17.6	3.0	17,722,672	2,782,440
Completed	14.8	2.1	14,903,156	1,947,708
Attempted only	2.8	0.9	2,819,516	834,732
Total physical assault	51.9	66.4	52,261,743	61,584,672
Threw something	14.0	22.4	14,097,580	20,775,552
Pushed, grabbed, shoved	30.6	43.5	30,813,282	40,345,380
Pulled hair	19.0	17.9	19,132,430	16,601,892
Slapped, hit	43.0	53.7	43,299,710	49,805,676
Kicked, bit	8.9	15.2	8,962,033	14,097,696
Choked, tried to drown	7.7	3.9	753,669	3,617,172
Hit with object	21.2	34.7	21,347,764	32,183,556
Beat up	14.1	15.5	14,198,277	14,375,940
Threatened with gun	6.2	13.1	6,243,214	12,149,988
Threatened with knife	5.8	16.1	5,840,426	14,932,428
Used gun	2.6	5.1	2,618,122	4,730,148
Used knife	3.5	9.6	3,524,395	8,903,808
Rape and/or physical assault	55.0	66.8	55,383,350	61,955,664

[a](n = number of people surveyed)

[b](Estimated number of men and women in the United States age 18 years and older)

Source: National Violence Against Women Survey, Centers for Disease Control and Prevention, 1998.

How does that violence affect a developing mind? The answer seems to be that such children become desensitized to violence—they get used to it. A 2003 study of youths in Los Angeles published in the *Journal of Education* found that children who live with violence have poorer grades in school, less energy, and lower expectations for themselves than other children. Young victims of violence tended to be more aggressive and less able to concentrate on schoolwork. The results of a 2000 study published in the *Journal of Consulting and Clinical Psychology* suggest that youthful victims of violence have trouble controlling their emotions, easily become angry, and experience difficulty making and keeping friends.

A violent upbringing continues to affect children as they grow older. A 2008 report in the *Journal of Family Issues* provides additional evidence that violence is transmitted between generations. The authors of the study found that abused children were more likely as adults to also abuse their own children. One controversial finding is those children who experienced severe abuse were less likely as adults to abuse their own children. The authors admit to being surprised by this finding and believe more research is needed to determine the reasons behind it. The finding could be a fluke, due to the way the study was conducted, or severe abuse may have instilled on the victims that this type of behavior is unacceptable, thereby reducing the odds that they will abuse their own children.

Thirty years ago, when family violence first became a public concern, it was a very difficult aspect of American life to research. Today, it remains difficult for researchers to even define the scope of problem. Nearly every study on child abuse, domestic violence, and elder abuse cites a lack of firm figures because of underreporting. Whether from shame or because they can't believe they are actually in an abusive situation, many people keep silent when they are in trouble.

See also: Legal Interventions; Sexual Violence; Social Costs of Violence; Violent Behavior, Causes of

FURTHER READING

Brown, Isobel. *Domestic Crime.* Broomall, Pa: Mason Crest Publishers, 2003.

Dutton, Donald G. *Rethinking Domestic Violence.* Vancouver: University of British Columbia Press, 2007.

■ FIGHT OR FLIGHT RESPONSE

An instinctive reaction to danger or stress. The fight or flight response is a throwback to prehistoric times, when a split second could mean the difference between life and death, between being fed or feeding a predator. Today, this instinct plays a part in the way humans respond to conflict, frustration, and anxiety.

Few people encounter hungry wolves or bears today. They may, however, have to deal with an exam in literature class, a basketball game against a rival school, or an attempt to persuade a parent to reconsider a curfew. Among the bodily responses that accompany these experiences are a racing heart, sweaty palms, and heavy breathing. More extreme situations may produce dizziness or nausea. All of these reactions are normal, part of the fight or flight response.

When someone encounters a **stressor**—an item or situation that causes stress—the body prepares itself either to meet the challenge head-on or to come up with an escape plan and avoid it.

THE BIOLOGICAL RESPONSE

The fight or flight response does not involve the higher thinking parts of the brain. It comes from the **autonomic nervous system** (ANS), in the primitive parts of the brain, the spinal cord, and nerves in the chest area. The ANS runs functions that usually do not require conscious control, like digesting food, the pumping of the heart, and breathing.

When stress is detected, the ANS "revs up" body functions. Chemicals called **hormones** flood the system, preparing the body for sudden, extreme exertion. Among these body chemicals are epinephrine, known as the fear hormone, and norepinephrine, the anger hormone. A rush of emotions overpowers the thinking parts of the brain, which may explain why some students "melt down" on major tests. They literally cannot access the information they studied. Instinctive response may be necessary in a physical crisis, where action is needed rather than thoughtful debate. Unfortunately, modern sources of stress (like tests, job interviews, or traffic problems) cannot be resolved by running away or lashing out in anger.

In a physical sense, everyone reacts to stressful situations in the same way. Why are some people able to deal with the stress, while others resort to violence? The answer lies in the ability to manage the degree of anxiety connected with the stress.

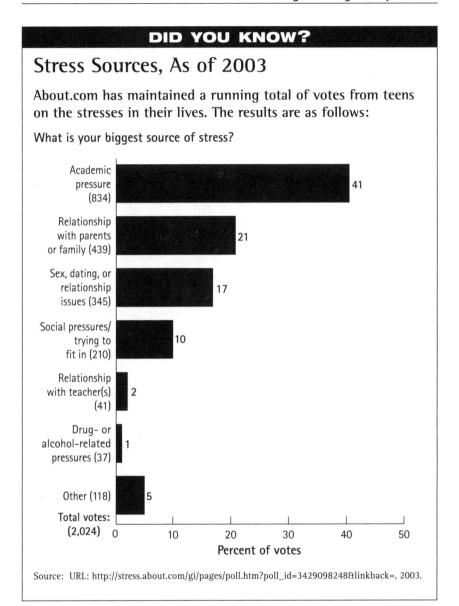

DID YOU KNOW?

Stress Sources, As of 2003

About.com has maintained a running total of votes from teens on the stresses in their lives. The results are as follows:

What is your biggest source of stress?

Academic pressure (834): 41
Relationship with parents or family (439): 21
Sex, dating, or relationship issues (345): 17
Social pressures/ trying to fit in (210): 10
Relationship with teacher(s) (41): 2
Drug- or alcohol-related pressures (37): 1
Other (118): 5
Total votes: (2,024)

Percent of votes

Source: URL: http://stress.about.com/gi/pages/poll.htm?poll_id=3429098248&linkback=, 2003.

THE HARDY PERSONALITY

In his 1999 address to the American Psychological Association conference, Salvatore Maddi reflected on his 20 years of researching what is called the **hardy personality.** Maddi and his colleagues discovered that three mental attitudes determine how well a person is likely to handle stress. These are commitment, control, and challenge.

An individual's level of commitment demonstrates a willingness to be involved with other people rather than being alone. Connections to others and to the world around him or her can help an individual handle stress in a more positive fashion. Control, says Maddi, involves "struggling to have an influence on outcomes." Those who maintain control do not respond passively or feel powerless. Finally, accepting the challenge of day-to-day living reflects a desire to learn from experiences rather than taking the easy way out or letting fear of a possible failure stop one from trying. Today these attitudes are referred to as the **three Cs of hardiness.**

The notion of hardiness helps explain why some people handle stress well, while others resort to violence. Individuals who believe they have some say in the outcome of life events and are willing to accept both success and failure are more likely to handle stress well. For some people violence becomes an expression of fear. They may dread the uncertainty of a situation or fear that it is beyond control. Acting out becomes a way to prevent change. Developing the three Cs of hardiness can help to reduce levels of anxiety, and, in turn, reduce the degree of violence. A major step in the right direction is working to change one's outlook or mood.

ENHANCING YOUR MOOD

When someone is observed acting in an aggressive way, people often comment that he or she "is in a bad mood." One's mood is a result of the complicated interaction of all body systems. However, according to a series of California-based research studies published in the *Journal of Personality and Social Psychology* in 1994, people can do a variety of things to enhance their mood. The California researchers defined a good mood as a high state of energy combined with a low state of tension. Unfortunately, many everyday events cause stress and lower one's energy. The California researchers found that people have the means to change their mood.

Mental approaches

- **Communication.** Most participants in the California studies reported that sharing what was bothering them with another person helped to restore a positive mood. Calling someone, sitting down to talk, or just being

See also: Road Rage; Violent Behavior, Causes of

FURTHER READING
Casey, Carolyn. *Conflict Resolution: The Win–Win Situation.* Berkeley Heights, N.J.: Enslow Publishers, 2001.
Ursiny, Tim. *The Coward's Guide to Conflict: Empowering Solution for Those Who Would Rather Run Away Than Fight.* Naperville, Ill.: Sourcebooks, Inc., 2003.

■ GANG VIOLENCE

The violent behaviors of a group of people, usually young, who often band together for criminal purposes. Gangs are marked by an organized structure, criminal behavior as a focus of activity, and the use of symbols or rituals to reflect members' affiliation.

Gang activity is often violent because gangs commonly engage in lawbreaking, such as robbery, shaking down local businesses, car theft, weapons violations, and selling drugs.

Another source of violence is conflict with other gangs. As gangs develop, they usually stake out an area as their territory, or **turf**. Depending on the number of members and the degree of organization, gang turfs can include an entire neighborhood or a smaller area such as a particular housing project, a strip mall, a school, or a park. Whatever the space, gang members consider it forbidden ground for members of other gangs. Intruders face physical attack or worse, which leads to retaliation and sometimes escalates to outright gang wars.

One way gang members carry on conflict is through **drive-by shootings,** murders committed when one gang member drives a car past a group of rivals while another fires a weapon into the crowd. Such attacks often result in the death or injury of innocent bystanders.

THE CHANGING FACE OF GANGS

According to a 1998 article in the *Juvenile Justice Bulletin,* writers have been describing gang-like behavior among young men in American cities since 1783. Social scientists did not begin to study street gangs until the 1920s, and gangs did not become a concern of the general public until the 1950s. Movies like *The Wild One* portrayed motorcycle gangs, while *The Blackboard Jungle* showed an urban, school-centered gang. *West Side Story,* a Broadway musical turned hit film, featured an urban gang war.

In the 1950s, gang members were considered "juvenile delinquents." People expected them to outgrow gang behavior. However, many gangs have not faded away. The Vice Kings in Chicago were organized in the 1950s and still recruit members today. Since the 1980s, a number of gangs have also enlarged their geographic spread, starting operations in other cities. The 1998 article in *Juvenile Justice Bulletin* points out that in the 1980s, gang membership changed, with a greater number of both older and younger members. Gangs began to have *veteranos,* members who have belonged to the gang for 18 years or more.

The 1980s also marked major media exposure for gangs and the gang lifestyle. Coverage of the ongoing street war between the Crips and the Bloods in Los Angeles placed those two organizations center stage, making their blue and red identifying colors known nation-wide. In some areas, local gangs began adopting similar names and colors.

In discussions about colors, tattoos, and graffiti, people often overlook a number of groups. **Skinheads,** groups that promote racial supremacy, are also considered gangs. These young people are looked on as the "frontline warriors" for organizations like the Ku Klux Klan and the White Aryan Resistance. Left-wing gangs, like Straight Edge, vandalize fur and furniture stores in the name of animal rights.

TEENS SPEAK

One Shot from the Edge

Neal is 19 years old. He ran with a gang for three years.

"So there I was, walking down the street with a gun down my pants. My gang, the Playboys, sent me out to kill a guy from the Kings. He'd shot some of our brothers while they were on the way to mess up a Kings' party. One of our guys had to ditch the machete he was carrying before they took him to the emergency room."

Neal shrugs as he looks back. "I realized this was get-ting pretty heavy. I'd been with the gang for three years, since my family got—what do they call it? Dysfunctional. Dad split, Mom worked, and I started hanging with the Playboys.

"While I was looking for that guy from the Kings, the gun I was carrying just got bigger and heavier. I was tight with one guy who'd shot somebody. They'd dissed him in the street, and the other brothers kept dogging him until he took out a gun and shot the guy."

His face gets very tight. "We all ran, but my buddy got caught and ended up being put away for a long time. I hear he curses the day he ever carried a gun.

"Maybe it's lucky I was alone. If the brothers had been dogging me, I might have gone through with it. Instead, I ended up throwing the gun in a sewer. I went home, started dressing like a regular person—no colors. I've got a job, and I'm working for my GED."

Neal shakes his head. "Now I've got a shot at having a life—instead of having it end because I shot somebody, or somebody shot me."

ACCEPTANCE BY A GANG

Why would a young person embrace a violent and dangerous lifestyle? Often they live in dangerous and violent neighborhoods. In the *Juvenile Justice Bulletin* article, many gang members cited protection as a major reason for joining. According to the Violence Prevention Institute, there are several reasons children and teenagers join gangs. Reasons include developing a sense of identity, seeking protection, looking for fellowship (a bond similar to that found in families), and being coerced or intimidated.

Many gangs are good at convincing potential members to join. The Comprehensive Community Reanimation Process, published by Urban Dynamics, Inc., spells out many of the techniques used by gangs to recruit members. Often, current members will tell tales of glory and spectacular lifestyles to convince young people that the gang is the place to be. The image of driving an expensive car with lots of money in one's pocket and an arsenal of weapons in the trunk has a powerful lure for some teens even if they suspect that the picture the gang paints is untrue or unrealistic. A sense of obligation can be yet another strong influence on young people. Essentially, gang members say, "If I do you a favor, then you owe me, and my 'fee' is your loyalty to the gang."

The media also plays a part in encouraging young people to join gangs. As early as 1961, big-budget movies portrayed gang involvement. While the dancing gang members in *West Side Story* may seem old-fashioned to today's young audiences, the characters have cool nicknames, hang out at a local store, and do not go to school. To some people, that sounds like fun. Films such as *South Central* and *New Jack City* show a harder-edged view of the drugs and violence associated with gangs, but still present the tight connection among gang members in a favorable light. For a young person with a difficult home life, the notion of gaining a family may outweigh the drug and violence issues.

THERE ARE NO GANGS HERE . . . ARE THERE?

The majority of young people who join gangs feel cut off from their family or their community, and the sense of belonging to a group that will love them and protect them is powerful. This disconnected feeling used to be attributed to poor family structures in the inner city. Therefore, gang activity has long been considered an urban problem. It was thought that only big cities like Los Angeles, New York, and Chicago had gang problems, not small towns or rural areas. Today, law enforcement officers and researchers are aware that gangs are no longer an urban problem. For many reasons, young adults feel alienated. Membership in a gang has become a way for many of them to find security.

In the 1995 book *The American Street Gang,* author M. W. Klein shared his research on gang growth. In 1960, only 58 cities reported gang activity. By 1980, 179 cities reported gangs, and by 1992, that figure had risen to 769 cities.

In 2001, the *Report on the Growth of Youth Gang Problems in the United States, 1970–1998* was issued by the Office of Juvenile Justice and Delinquency Prevention. According to this report, 201 cities reported gang activity in the 1970s. That figure rose to 468 cities in the 1980s, and to 1,487 cities by the mid-1990s. The report also viewed gang growth in terms of the counties affected. In 1970, the counties with gang activity represented 35.6 percent of the total population of the United States. By 1995, 77.9 percent of the population lived in counties with gang activity.

The National Youth Gang Survey issued by the Department of Justice estimated that there were more than 27,000 gangs in 2007, with members in excess of 788,000. The New York Police Department's

---

DID YOU KNOW?

Risk Factors at Ages 10–12 for Gang Membership

Potential Childhood Risk Factor	Percent of Youths Who Join Gangs*
Neighborhood	
Availability of marijuana	30
Neighborhood youths in trouble	26
Low neighborhood attachment	20
Family	
Poverty (low household income)	23
One parent in home	21
One parent and other adults in home	25
No parents in home	24
Parental alcohol intake	15
Sibling antisocial behavior	22
Poor family management	21
Parental pro-violent attitudes	26
Low attachment to parents	20
School	
Low academic aspirations	20
Low school commitment	21
Low school attachment	23
Low academic achievement in elementary school	28
Identified as learning disabled	36
Peer	
Association with peers who engage in problem behaviors	26

* Percentage of youths joining a gang among youths who had scored in the worst quarter on the risk factor at ages 10–12

Source: Office of Juvenile Justice and Delinquency Prevention, 1999.

gang intelligence unit reported that gangs were operating 95 percent of the large cities in the United States and 88 percent of the smaller ones.

Speaking to the 1996 conference of the Violence Intervention and Prevention Institute (VIP), Michael Walker of the Partnership for a Safer Cleveland discussed conditions that seem to foster gang growth. Any region where factories and other businesses are closing and the unemployment rate is disproportionately high has an increased chance of seeing gang activity develop.

Another major change in gangs involves girls. A 1998 article in *Crime & Justice,* an annual review of research, reports that it is difficult to get an accurate picture of the degree of female involvement in gangs. Police tend to underreport data on female gangs. As a result, police statistics suggest that women are responsible for only about 5 percent of gang activity. However, the article notes that additional information produced by researchers suggests that up to one-half of all gang members are girls.

GANGS AND SCHOOLS

The culture of many high schools is a good fit for gang activity. High schools are filled with young teens trying to fit in, to join a welcoming group to which they can relate—exactly what gang members tell them a gang can offer. As a result, in communities where illegal drug sales are high, the school may become a battleground with gangs fighting to corner the market.

Based on what is known about why youths join gangs, schools can discourage gang membership by creating an environment where students feel welcome and educators help students feel as though they belong. Speaking on gang prevention at the 1996 VIP Institute, Walker identified the following as important lessons that should affect the way schools are run:

- Focus activities on nine- to 12-year-olds, before they have an opportunity to join a gang and while they are not yet adolescents

- Start programs early and continue them throughout a child's years in school

- Ask young people to play a role in the development of activities and policies that help teach and reinforce the skills that discourage gang activity

- Remember young people are individuals—they do not all think, act, or behave in unison and should not be treated as though they do
- Get families involved
- Encourage local business leaders and organizations to assist the school in providing activities that meet the needs of students
- Keep school-based activities connected to local organizations. Resources can be pooled and children can be more easily networked in the community through preexisting relationships

A 1997 article in the *Journal of Gang Research* argues that schools need to recognize the signs that gangs are being formed in order to prevent their activity in the school. Researchers suggest that schools start by identifying students who may fit the gang member profile.

Which students show signs of needing the type of support a gang claims to provide? In his 1995 book, *The American Street Gang*, M. W. Klein suggests that gang members are not very different from their non-gang peers. However, gang members do tend to demonstrate some of the following attributes to a greater extent when contrasted with non-gang youths:

- Difficulty with school work, often having lower than normal IQs
- Poor impulse control
- A marked tendency toward aggressiveness and physical prowess
- Inadequate social skills
- An enhanced need, or desire, for belonging
- An enhanced need, or desire, for status and recognition
- A boring, uninvolved lifestyle in which episodes of excitement are sought and valued
- A weak or nonexistent attachment to adult control systems
- A lack of structure to develop personal and social identity

Once school officials have determined which students are most vulnerable to gang influence, they also need to watch for symbols of gang membership. Are distinctive patterns of color showing up in some student circles? Has graffiti appeared on the school grounds? School personnel should be trained to recognize how gang development looks. Most importantly, the staff needs to enforce school rules in a consistent way. Officials also need to work with students to develop communication and conflict resolution skills to reduce violent outcomes in conflict situations.

Gangs have appeared in all 50 states, in almost every racial and ethnic group, in a variety of social and economic situations, in large cities and small towns. Experience has shown the problems associated with intervention–trying to get young people out of gangs once they have become established is difficult. Yet preventing gangs from organizing in the first place is an important step in reducing the threat of violence for young people in their homes, neighborhoods, and schools.

Q & A

Question: I don't want to be in a gang any longer. How can I get out?

Answer: With some gangs, it's easy to get in and get out. With others, getting out can be difficult and even dangerous. The National Alliance of Gang Investigators Associations offers this advice:

- Never tell the gang that you plan to leave—you may be beaten or even killed.
- Stop hanging around with gang friends and find something else to do—sports, clubs, school or family activities.
- Stop dressing and talking like a gang member.
- Become good at making excuses—when gang members call, you have to be either away or busy doing something else. With luck, this will allow you to "fade away" from the gang.
- Find people who will believe in you and will help you by offering support and good advice.

Leaving a gang may be a struggle, but it will let you escape from a dead-end street and win your life back.

Fact Or Fiction?

Being in a gang protects me while I live in a violent neighborhood.

The Facts: It might seem like a good idea to have a gang to watch one's back in a dangerous neighborhood. The National Alliance of Gang Investigators Associations points out, however, that becoming a gang member makes a person a target for rival gangs. Gang members face an increased risk of being injured or killed. The simple act of leaving their neighborhoods exposes them to danger. Even if they succeed in leaving a gang, their former rivals can still make dangerous enemies.

See also: Assault and Bullying; Media and Violence; School Violence; Teens and Violence

FURTHER READING

Cozic, Charles P., ed. *Gangs: Opposing Viewpoints.* San Diego: Greenhaven Press, 1996.

Hagedorn, John M. *A World of Gangs: Armed Young Men and Gangsta Culture.* Minneapolis: University of Minnesota Press, 2008.

■ GUN USE

See: Criminals and Violent Activity; School Violence; Weapons of Violence

■ HATE CRIMES

According to the U.S. Department of Justice, violence intended to hurt and intimidate someone because of his or her race, ethnicity, national origin, religion, sexual orientation, or disability. Examples of hate crimes in the news in the past years include the slashing of car tires in a predominantly Jewish neighborhood; a Sikh restaurant owner being taunted as a terrorist, then beaten because he wore a turban; an African American dragged to his death after being chained to a pickup truck; and a gay man severely beaten, tied to a fence, and left to die.

No two human beings are exactly alike. People differ in countless ways from one another, including interests, abilities, skin color, religion, sexual preference, neighborhood, and family wealth. For some people, those differences become a way of distinguishing themselves from others.

According to many psychologists, although it is natural to see oneself as an individual and view others as representatives of groups. **Stereotypes** are offensive. They are more than a label or judgment about an individual based on the characteristics of a group. Stereotyping reduces individuals to categories. Therefore stereotyping can lead to **prejudice** and **discrimination**. The word *prejudice* means "prejudgment." People prejudge when they have an opinion about another person based on his or her membership in a particular group. A prejudice attaches value to differences to the benefit of one's own group and at the expense of other groups. Discrimination occurs when prejudices are translated into actions. When those actions become violent, they are considered hate crimes. Not every stereotype results in discrimination, but all stereotypes tend to divide a society into "us" and "them."

In their article on hate crimes in the *Encyclopedia of Peace, Violence, and Conflict,* Northwestern University professors Jack Levin and Jack McDevitt point out that since the 1980s, some members of majority groups have viewed efforts to end discrimination as challenges to their own status. These individuals view dramatic increases in interfaith and interracial dating and marriage as a threat. They are also troubled by newly arrived immigrants from Latin America and Asia. They are uncomfortable with racial integration in their neighborhoods, schools, and workplaces. They are outraged by the number of gay men and lesbians who have "come out" and, in many cases, begun organizing for equal status in their communities. Hate crimes are the responses of certain members of the majority to such perceived threats.

THE MENTALITY BEHIND THE HATRED

Many would like to believe that the people who commit hate crimes are hate-crazed extremists. Research at the University of California, Los Angeles, reveals that of 1,459 hate crimes committed in the Los Angeles area from 1994 to 1995, fewer than 5 percent of those responsible belonged to organized hate groups. Most offenders were otherwise law-abiding young people who saw little wrong with their actions. Alcohol and drugs sometimes fueled hate crimes, but in general, people who commit hate crimes believe that the society as a whole gives them permission to attack certain groups.

In a 1997 Congressional Briefing on hate crimes, psychologist Karen Franklin discussed a study of 500 people from the San Francisco area. About 10 percent of the subjects admitted physical violence or threats against people whom they believed to be gay. Another 24 percent reported antigay name-calling. Among men, 18 percent admitted to acts of violence or threats of violence, with 32 percent resorting to name-calling. An additional 30 percent stated that they would react aggressively if a gay person flirted with or propositioned them.

The study examined the motives in antigay crimes and found four:

- Self-defense. Attackers saw sexual propositions as aggressive acts by gay predators.
- Ideology. Attackers acted from negative beliefs about homosexuality, often seeing themselves as defending traditional values.
- Thrill-seeking. Attacks resulted from a desire for excitement or to feel strong.
- Peer dynamics. Attackers joined others to prove their toughness or heterosexuality to friends.

At the same briefing, Donald Green, an expert on hate crimes, noted that such crimes often occur when minorities move into previously all-white areas. The offenders frequently justify their actions as defending a rapidly disappearing traditional way of life. Green also discussed this "defended neighborhood" excuse in a 1997 study for Yale University's Institution for Social and Political Studies.

The Encyclopedia of Peace, Violence, and Conflict points out that hate crimes are crimes with a message. That message is aimed not only at the victim but also at people *like* the victim. In fact, a 1995 study of hate crimes in Boston reported in *Klanwatch Intelligence Report* showed that 66 percent of the people committing the crimes did not know the victims. A rock through a window is not merely an act of vandalism, but a notice that an entire group is not welcome in a community, a workplace, or school.

Hate messages also go out over the media. In the book *Waves of Rancour: Tuning in the Radical Right,* authors Robert Hilliard and Michael Keith point out that more than 1,000 groups—usually calling themselves patriotic—denounce immigration, racial integration, and warn of "an international Jewish conspiracy" to take over the world, spearheaded by control of American finance and Hollywood. This propaganda is promoted in high-tech ways, from CDs for skinhead rock bands to the Internet. Entering "Jew" in the popular search engine Google gives an address for an anti-Semitic Web site in the top 10 responses.

Even the mainstream media can spark hate crimes. When a New York City talk-radio host launched a particularly sharp attack on immigrants from India who were moving into a New Jersey town in 1996, numerous ethnic slurs were spray-painted on Indian-owned homes and businesses the next day. Shots were even fired through the windows of one home owned by recent immigrants.

WHO ARE THE VICTIMS?

The victims of hate crimes in the United States are groups that are seen as different from the majority. Racial and religious minorities, homosexuals, and immigrants are often targeted. According to the Federal Bureau of Investigation (FBI), there were an estimated 7,624 incidents of hate crimes in 2007, involving 9,535 victims. Almost 51 percent of these incidents were racially motivated, while 18.4 percent were motivated by religion.

In 2001, 9,730 hate crimes were reported. Part of the reason for the higher number was a surge in anti-Islamic crimes after the terrorist attacks on New York City and Washington, D.C., in 2001. From 28 attacks on Muslims in 2000, the number rose to 481 in 2001.

While more agencies now take part in the program, it still does not cover all hate crimes. Police departments differ in defining a hate crime and recording these crimes. A 1997 Department of Justice (DOJ) report, *A Policymaker's Guide to Hate Crimes,* suggests that crimes may be underreported. In cases of attacks on gays, many, especially those who have not "come out," are fearful of reporting an attack. Immigrants, especially those who have entered the country illegally or come from a country where the police are seen as the enemy, fear deportation if they report a hate crime.

According to the Anti-Defamation League, in 2007, there were 1,460 cases of anti-Semitic violence. This includes 699 acts of vandalism and 761 acts of harassment. Harassment is a broad category, including both physical and verbal assaults against institutions and individuals. Data from the FBI indicate there were 1,628 victims of antireligious hate crimes. This includes the 1,128 victims of anti-

Semitic hate crimes. The most common type of crime was vandalism and destruction of property.

Some suggest that advocacy groups may tend to overcount, but even the DOJ believes that its figures underrepresent the problem of hate crimes.

WHAT CAN BE DONE?

Hate crimes are, by definition, crimes. Whether someone attacks a person to steal a wallet or because the individual is different, the perpetrator is still guilty of a crime. Most states have laws against hate crimes, often adding extra penalties, such as additional prison time, for crimes motivated by hate. These laws have been challenged in the courts, but the Supreme Court has upheld the concept.

The effort to legislate against hate-inciting speech has proven more controversial. Canada and many European countries, including Britain and Germany, have laws that ban hate speech. The United States, however, protects such speech in the First Amendment to the Constitution.

State laws have tried to attack hate speech by banning **fighting words**—forms of expression designed to enrage listeners and incite violence—from radio and television broadcasts. The courts have struck down most of these laws, because the language of these laws is too vague.

Criminologist Jack Levin took a more concrete view in a 2003 speech to students and faculty at Rhode Island College. He pointed out that most hate crimes are not committed by members of organized hate groups, but by young people who live nearby. Many people are bystanders during a hate crime. By not speaking out, they silently give permission to the criminals.

Levin challenged his audience to stand up for the people who have been targeted. He ended his speech by telling his listeners, "Please don't forget where hate begins, and that is in the silence of ordinary people."

See also: Gang Violence; Media and Violence

FURTHER READING

Ehrlich, Howard J. *Hate Crimes and Ethnoviolence: The History, Current Affairs, and Future of Discrimination in America.* Boulder, Colo.: Westview Press, 2009.

Levin, Jack, and Jack McDevitt. "Hate Crimes." In *Encyclopedia of Peace, Violence, and Conflict.* New York: Academic Press, 1999.

■ HOMICIDE

The killing of one human being by another. In the eyes of the law, homicide is not always a crime. According to *Black's Law Dictionary*, the word *homicide* is a legally neutral term. Although **murder** and **manslaughter** are crimes, a person may kill in self-defense or to stop an escaping criminal. Homicide is also justifiable if taking a life is a part of one's duty as a prison executioner, for example. **Excusable homicide** occurs when the killing has no criminal intent. For example, a person who kills an attacker has committed excusable homicide.

Unlawful killing is called **felonious** or **criminal homicide**. Both murder and manslaughter fall into this category. To convict a person of a murder requires proof of planning and intent to do harm. It has to be a "willful" act. Manslaughter is murder without intent. Manslaughter can be voluntary, such as a deadly fistfight, or involuntary, such as an accident caused by a speeding car. Like murder, both voluntary and involuntary manslaughter are considered criminal homicides.

Fact Or Fiction?

Murders are the most committed crimes.

The Facts: Murder may seem to be the most common crime, if you read mystery novels or watch films and TV dramas. However, murders make up the smallest category of violent crimes in the FBI's Uniform Crime Reporting Program. In 2007, law enforcement agencies across the country reported 16,929 murders. In the same period, they reported 90,427 forcible rapes and 445,125 robberies. Cases of aggravated assault—attacks with a weapon or attempts at great bodily harm—totaled 855,856.

THE EXTENT OF CRIMINAL HOMICIDE

According to a fact sheet on leading causes of death from the Centers for Disease Control and Prevention, homicide was responsible for 7.1 percent of American deaths in 2003. The report also noted that homicide was "not ranked as one of the top ten leading causes of death, but a leading source of death in certain demographic groups."

In 2007, the Federal Bureau of Investigation received supplemental homicide data on 14,831 murders. This data allows the FBI to provide more details on the victims, offenders, and events surrounding the homicides. Of the 14,831 murders for which additional information was provided, 7,316 victims (49.3 percent) were black. The data also

show that 6,463 homicide offenders were black, which is 37.9 percent of all homicide offenders. Yet, it is estimated that blacks make up only 13.5 percent of the total population, indicating that African Americans are overrepresented in homicide statistics.

When homicide occurs to the most vulnerable in society, it tends to stir people's emotions. **Infanticide** is the murder of children under the age of five, while **eldercide** is the murder of persons 65 and older. Infanticide is the only category of homicide that increased during the 1990s, although it did decline slightly toward the end of the decade. Approximately 600 children under five years of age were killed in 2000, over half by a parent. Eldercide accounted for about 5 percent of all homicides in 2000. The rate of homicide of persons over 65 years of age has been declining since the early 1980s.

Q & A

Question: Who is most likely to want to murder me—someone I know or a stranger?

Answer: After examining Department of Justice statistics from 1976 to 2002, researchers found that 13.9 percent of murderers were strangers to their victims. In 6.9 percent of the cases, the murderer was the victim's spouse—a husband or wife. An additional 7.8 percent of murders were committed by some other family member, while 4.4 percent were committed by a boyfriend or girlfriend. Acquaintances were responsible for 32.6 percent of the murders studied. This classification includes friends, coworkers, fellow students, and people met at parties or events. The "acquaintance" tag is rather vague—it can also refer to drug dealers and their customers and even cover the relationship between a cab driver and a passenger. In 34.4 percent of the murders, the relationship between the victim and the murderer remained undetermined.

REASONS PEOPLE KILL

Among the facts and figures presented in the *2009 Statistical Abstract of the United States* is a listing of circumstances for murders that occurred the previous year. A good proportion of homicides—16.3 percent—were connected with felonies: 6.9 percent involved robbery, 5.3 percent involved drugs, and 0.2 percent involved rapes. The largest single cause for murder was disagreements. Disputes, whether over property, money, romance, or other reasons, accounted for 48.5 percent of killings. Other motives were cited in 20.0 percent of the cases, while the circumstances for 34.8 percent of murders are unknown.

Facts and figures seem inadequate in explaining *why* people commit homicide. In 1999, two students at Columbine High School in Colorado killed 13 people and then themselves. Responding to the murders, the American Psychological Association and MTV developed a program on school violence called Warning Signs. The program materials point to a number of reasons for the rise in violence and murder:

- Easy availability of guns. The United States has some of the weakest gun laws in the world. Although events like the Columbine massacre have occurred in other countries, only in the United States are large numbers of weapons so easily available.

- Online availability of information on explosives. Before the Internet, such information was difficult to obtain, even in libraries. Today, that information is available with the click of a mouse.

- The breakdown of the nuclear family. The increasing divorce rate and the blending of families seem to make it harder for children to find role models that can help them learn how to resolve conflicts. Children learn from what they see, not what they hear.

- Violence on television and in movies. How many murders does the average person witness each week? The average TV watcher sees several during the course of a week. While violence may add excitement to television and movies, it also presents behaviors that some young people try to imitate.

- The absence of a moral compass. In the past, young people had access to religious groups and organizations like the Boys Scouts and Girl Scouts that provided moral guidance. Today far fewer young people are exposed to these influences.

- Both parents working. Many families need the income from the work of both parents. However, when both parents work, children have far more unsupervised time than was true for past generations. Most children do not build bombs in the basement, but decreased parental involvement offers the opportunity.

- The breakdown of neighborhoods and communities. At one time, people tended to know everyone who lived on their block and many participated in community activities. Today families tend to spend more time apart from their community. Teenagers who do not feel connected to the community are more likely to act out in destructive ways.

- The tendency of teens to form cliques. Teen movies have turned the social structure in high schools—jocks and popular kids on top, others on the fringe—into a stereotype. Unfortunately, the stereotype has some basis in fact. Conflicts among groups within a school have always existed, but today they are more violent, often involving weapons instead of fists.

- Healthy teen rebellion getting out of hand. Teenagers struggle to become their own person, in part by rebelling against their parents. However, this normal process can go too far. If rebellion cuts all lines of communication between parents and teens, everyone suffers.

Homicides have decreased with the general decline of crime rates in recent years. However, 2006 statistics compiled by the Centers for Disease Control and Prevention on the top 10 causes of death for Americans still point out some disturbing facts. In the 10- to 14-year-old age range, homicide was third on the list. For the 15- to 19-year-old group, homicide was the second-highest cause of death.

See also: Gang Violence; Media and Violence; School Violence; Teens and Violence; Weapons of Violence

FURTHER READING

Ewing, Charles Patrick. *When Kids Kill.* New York: HarperCollins, 1995.

Shon, Phillip C., and Dragan Milovanovic. *Serial Killers: Understanding Lust Murder.* Durham, N.C.: Carolina Academic Press, 2006.

■ INCARCERATION

Confinement to prison or jail of individuals charged with or convicted of crimes. Incarceration is designed to keep offenders out of the community and deter them from committing future crimes.

The United States has a long history of incarcerating people. In colonial times, two prisons helped shape the country's approach to incarceration—the Eastern State Penitentiary in Pennsylvania and the Auburn Prison in upper New York state. These institutions helped shape the minimum, medium, maximum, and super-maximum security prisons that currently exist. Although prisons at least temporarily keep offenders out of the community, evidence suggests they do little to deter people from committing crimes.

BRIEF HISTORY OF INCARCERATION

Facilities designed to hold suspected and convicted criminals have existed for centuries. When looking at modern jails and prisons in the United States, there were two early prisons that defined the country's approach to incarceration. Eastern State Penitentiary, located in Pennsylvania, opened in 1829, although construction was not completed until 1836. At the time, the prison was the largest in the country. It followed the principle of solitary confinement, with only one inmate per cell. Cells were designed to be large enough to allow an inmate to have a work station and an exercise yard. The cells also had toilets and showers. The idea was to keep inmates completely separate. This model became known as the separate system. There were three problems with this type of system that became evident immediately. Prisons using this model would have to be extremely large in order to provide inmates with individual cells. Second, these prisons could not hold as many inmates as prisons built according to a different layout. Third, it was very expensive to build such a large facility.

In Auburn, New York, construction began on the Auburn Prison in 1816, with the first building being completed in approximately one year. By 1823, most of the facility had been built. The Auburn Prison was almost the opposite of the Eastern Penitentiary. Cells were much smaller, in some cases only a few feet wide by six to eight feet long. The Auburn model became known as the silent system. Inmates worked together; however, they were forbidden to speak. Whereas Eastern Penitentiary had to be spread out to enforce the separate system, Auburn Prison was taller, with cells located on several floors. As a result, more prisoners could be housed in less space. Inmates were

DID YOU KNOW?

People in U.S. Prisons or Jails

	Number of Inmates			Average annual change, 2000–2006 (%)	Percent change, 2006–2007 (%)
	2000	2006	2007		
Total inmates in custody[a]	1,937,482	2,258,983	2,293,157	2.6	1.5
Federal prisoners[b] (total)	140,064	190,844	197,285	5.3	3.4
Prisons	133,921	183,381	189,154	5.4	3.1
Federal facilities	124,540	163,118	165,975	4.6	1.8
Privately operated facilities	9,381	20,263	23,179	13.7	14.4
Community corrections centers[c]	6,143	7,463	8,131	3.3	9.0
State Prisoners	1,176,269	1,302,129	1,315,291	1.7	1.0
Inmates held in local jails	621,149	766,010	780,581	3.6	1.9
Incarceration rate[d]	684	751	756		

Note: Counts include all inmates held in public and private adult correctional facilities and in local jails.

[a]Total includes all inmates held in state or federal public facilities or in local jails. It does not include inmates held in U.S. territories, military facilities, U.S. Immigration and Customs Enforcement facilities, jails in Indian Country, and juvenile facilities.

[b]After 2001, responsibility for sentenced felons from the District of Columbia was transferred to the Federal Bureau of Prisons.

[c]Non-secure; privately operated community correction centers.

[d]The total number of inmates in custody per 100,000 U.S. residents.

Every year since 2000, the number of people incarcerated has increased. For every 100,000 people in the United States, 756 people are currently incarcerated. In all, at the end of 2006, there were more than 2 million people in prison or jail in the United States.

Source: *Prisoners in 2007.* Bureau of Justice Statistics, 2008.

forced to work, with prison officials making money by contracting inmate labor to companies. Auburn Prison became a model that was imitated across the country. Officials around the world also viewed the prison as an excellent facility.

TYPES OF PRISONS

Offenders convicted of a **felony** will serve time in a prison. Offenders convicted of lesser offenses, known as **misdemeanors,** will serve time in a jail, along with those who are still awaiting trial. The majority of inmates are housed in prisons. There are four types of prisons in the United States: minimum security, medium security, maximum security, and super-maximum security.

Minimum-security prisons hold the least dangerous offenders. A dormitory housing style is usually in place, and inmates are not closely supervised. Minimum-security prisons tend to offer more educational and rehabilitation programs to inmates. Many also have arrangements allowing inmates to work in the local community. Because these inmates pose the least amount of risk to the community, there typically is not much in the way of perimeter fencing at minimum security prisons, which exist at both the state and federal levels.

Medium-security prisons are more structured than minimum-security prisons. These prisons have more perimeter security systems in place to help prevent escapes and they place more restrictions on inmate behavior and privileges among inmates. Medium-security prisons offer a variety of work and rehabilitation programs. Whereas minimum-security prisons do not require a high ratio of guards to inmates, medium-security prisons employ more guards.

Maximum-security prisons tend to house violent offenders. At the federal level, these facilities are known as U.S. penitentiaries. They enforce a great deal of security: They may have several perimeter fences, often wrapped in barbed wire. Often they have prison towers, where guards keep watch on prisoners to prevent escape. Inside, cells are often opened from a remote room to help prevent rioting and escape. There is a high ratio of prison guards to inmates. Inmate behavior and activities are very controlled. These prisons tend to be considered dangerous because of the potential for violence among their inmates. There is only supposed to be one inmate per cell. However, due to prison overcrowding, it is common to find two and sometimes three inmates to a cell.

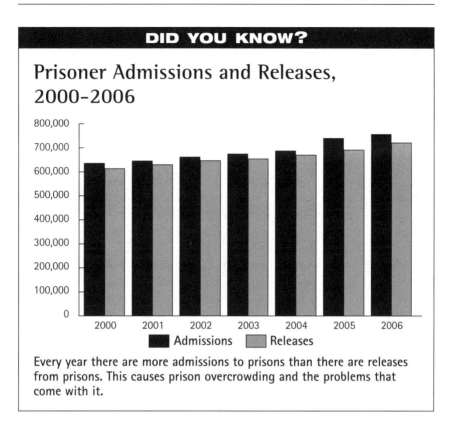

DID YOU KNOW?

Prisoner Admissions and Releases, 2000-2006

Every year there are more admissions to prisons than there are releases from prisons. This causes prison overcrowding and the problems that come with it.

Finally, there are the super-maximum, or supermax, security prisons. These prisons are designed to hold the most dangerous and violent offenders. Offenders who cause too many problems in a maximum-security prison may be transferred to a supermax facility. Other offenders may be directly imprisoned at a supermax facility, where inmates are completely isolated. There is little to no physical contact with prison staff. Inmates are not allowed to interact with other inmates. At best, inmates are allowed one hour in a highly secured outside area. If a prisoner has a visitor, he or she is separated by thick glass barriers. Inmates in a supermax facility are there for life.

SENTENCING OFFENDERS TO PRISON

Views differ as to how long offenders should remain in prison. Some believe that people charged with crimes should spend a specific amount of time in prison. State legislatures determine how long an

DID YOU KNOW?

Sentencing Guidelines for the State of Washington

Seriousness level	Offender score									
	0	1	2	3	4	5	6	7	8	9 or more
XVI	Life Sentence without Parole/Death Penalty									
XV	23y 4m	24y 4m	25y 4m	26y 4m	27y 4m	28y 4m	30y 4m	32y 10m	36y	40y
	240–320	250–333	261–347	271–361	281–374	291–388	312–416	338–450	370–493	411–548
XIV	14y 4m	15y 4m	16y 2m	17y	17y 11m	18y 9m	20y 5m	22y 2m	25y 7m	29y
	123–220	134–234	144–244	154–254	165–265	175–275	195–295	216–316	257–357	298–397
XIII	12y	13y	14y	15y	16y	17y	19y	21y	25y	29y
	123–164	134–178	144–192	154–205	165–219	175–233	195–260	216–288	257–342	298–397
XII	9y	9y 11m	10y 9m	11y 8m	12y 6m	13y 5m	15y 9m	17y 3m	20y 3m	23y 3m
	93–123	102–136	111–147	1 20–160	129–171	138–184	162–216	178–236	209–277	240–318
XI	7y 6m	8y 4m	9y 2m	9y 11m	10y 9m	11y 7m	14y 2m	15y 5m	17y 11m	20y 5m
	78–102	86–114	95–125	102 –136	111–147	120–158	146–194	159–211	185–245	210–280
X	5y	5y 6m	6y	6y 6m	7y	7y 6m	9y 6m	10y 6m	12y 6m	14y 6m
	51–68	57–75	62–82	67–89	72–96	77–102	98–130	108–144	129–171	149–198
IX	3y	3y 6m	4y	4y 6m	5y	5y 6m	7y 6m	8y 6m	10y 6m	12y 6m
	31–41	36–48	41–54	46–61	51–68	57–75	77–102	87–116	1 08–144	129–171

Offender Characteristics

DID YOU KNOW? (CONTINUED)

Offender Characteristics

VIII	2y / 21–27	2y 6m / 26–34	3y / 31–41	3y 6m / 36–48	4y / 41–54	4y 6m / 46–61	6y 6m / 67–89	7y 6m / 77–102	8y 6m / 87–116	10y 6m / 108–144
VII	18m / 15–20	2y / 21–27	2y 6m / 26–34	3y / 31–41	3y 6m / 36–48	4y / 41–54	5y 6m / 57–75	6y 6m / 67–89	7y 6m / 77–102	8y 6m / 87–116
VI	13m / 12+–14	18m / 15–20	2y / 21–27	2y 6m / 26–34	3y / 31–41	3y 6m / 36–48	4y 6m / 46–61	5y 6m / 57–75	6y 6m / 67–89	7y 6m / 77–102
V	9m / 6–12	13m / 12+–14	15m / 13–17	18m / 15–20	2y 2m / 22–29	3y 2m / 33–43	4y / 41–54	5y / 51–68	6y / 62–82	7y / 72–96
IV	6m / 3–9	9m / 6–12	13m / 12+–14	15m / 13–17	18m / 15–20	2y 2m / 22–29	3y 2m / 33–43	4y 2m / 43–57	5y 2m / 53–70	6y 2m / 63–84
III	2m / 1–3	5m / 3–8	8m / 4–12	11m / 9–12	14m / 12+–16	20m / 17–22	2y 2m / 22–29	3y 2m / 33–43	4y 2m / 43–57	5y / 51–68
II	0–90 days / days	4m / 2–6	6m / 3–9	8m / 4–12	13m / 12+–14	16m / 14–18	20m / 17–22	2y 2m / 22–29	3y 2m / 33–43	4y 2m / 43–57
I	0–60 days / days	3m / 2–5	4m / 2–6	5m / 3–8	8m / 4–12	13m / 12+–14	16m / 14–18	20m / 17–22	2y 2m / 22–29	2y 2m / 22–29

Most sentencing guidelines look like this chart. A judge takes both the severity of the offense (rows across) and offender characteristics, such as criminal history (columns down), into account when sentencing an offender to prison.

Source: *Adult Sentencing Manual 2008.* Washington State Sentencing Commission, 2008.

offender will be in jail based on the crimes committed. This is known as determinate sentencing.

Others believe that offenders should be subject to what is called an indeterminate sentence. By this approach, a state legislature sets a range of time that an offender may serve for a specific crime. There is a minimum amount of time and a maximum amount of time. The philosophy behind this approach is that each offender is different, and both the person and the crime should be taken into account when sentencing someone to prison. It also allows for rehabilitation opportunities. Inmates who work at bettering themselves may be released sooner than inmates who show no improvement. For example, the Utah State Sentencing Commission believes in indeterminate sentencing. In 2006, the commission wrote that a prisoner's "release is contingent on the individual nature of the crime committed, mitigating and aggravating circumstances associated with the criminal offense, past criminal history, the offender's conduct in the prison system, and proven amenability to rehabilitation over time."

Another type of sentence is the mandatory sentence. A mandatory sentence occurs when a legislature passes a law stating a certain type of crime requires, or mandates, a specific sentence. Even in states that use indeterminate sentencing, legislatures can require that certain crimes will carry a mandatory sentence. Every state has at least one mandatory sentencing law. Crimes committed with firearms often carry a mandatory sentence. Drug offenses will often carry such sentences.

A fourth type of sentencing is knowns as sentencing guidelines. This is used at the federal level and has been adopted by some states as well. States such as Washington, Oregon, Pennsylvania, Wisconsin, and Massachusetts use sentencing guidelines systems. This system combines indeterminate and determinate sentencing. Legislatures pass guidelines that judges and juries are supposed to follow. Guidelines take into account the seriousness of the crime and characteristics of the offender, such as prior arrests and convictions. A judge then follows the guidelines, which set the minimum and maximum sentence that can be imposed.

GOALS OF INCARCERATION

Punishment has several goals; however, only some are relevant to incarceration. One of the goals of sending people who break the law to jail is to incapacitate them. By removing offenders from the community, they are less likely to commit more crimes. This goal is temporary with regard to offenders who do not receive sentences of life in prison. At some point, offenders will be released back into the community.

Another goal of prison is to deter people from committing crimes. There are two forms of deterrence: general and specific. Specific deterrence causes a person either to be afraid of receiving a punishment or, having been punished, of being punished again. General deterrence occurs when people witness someone's punishment and do not engage in similar behavior out of fear of receiving the same punishment. Incarceration fulfills both types of deterrence. Ideally, people will not commit crimes that result in being incarcerated. Obviously that does not happen, so it is hoped that being incarcerated will deter criminals from committing future crimes.

A third goal of incarceration is retribution or vengeance. The goal is to inflict punishment on those who have hurt others. The phrase "an eye for an eye" best sums up this goal.

Of the three goals, deterrence is the most important in preventing additional crimes by inmates. Unfortunately, incarceration does not do a good job of deterring inmates. Data from the Bureau of Justice Statistics do not support the deterrence effect. A 2002 report from the BJS found that 67.5 percent of prisoners released in 1994 were rearrested within three years. The rearrest rate for property offenders was 73.8 percent; for drug offenders, it was 66.7 percent; and for violent offenders, it was 61.7 percent.

In a 2009 article published in *Law and Human Behavior*, the authors reported on a study on recidivism, or relapse into crime, of inmates released from minimum-, medium-, and maximum security prisons in Canada. Only 136 inmates agreed to participate in the study. The authors found that 36.8 percent of the inmates were returned to prison. About half of the inmates were returned to prison because they violated conditions of their release (parole). The others committed new offenses, with seven offenders being charged with a new violent crime.

A 2009 study was published in the *American Journal of Psychiatry* where the authors examined the role psychiatric disorders play in recidivism. The authors reviewed the records of 71,333 inmates in the Texas prison system. Inmates diagnosed with any psychiatric disorder were twice as likely as those without a disorder to have been in prison at least one other time. Inmates with psychiatric disorders were 2.4

times more likely than those without a disorder to have been incarcerated at least four times.

In an ideal system, people serving time in jail would be rehabilitated before being released. However, in reality, many individuals who enter jail or prison return to crime soon after they are released into society.

See also: Criminals and Violent Activity; Gang Violence; Rehabilitation and Treatment of Perpetrators.

FURTHER READING
Seghetti, Lisa M., and Alison M. Smith. *Federal Sentencing Guidelines: Background, Legal Analysis, and Policy Options.* Washington, D.C.: Congressional Research Service, 2007.
Useem, Bert, and Anne Morrison Piehl. *Prison State: The Challenge of Mass Incarceration.* New York: Cambridge University Press, 2008.

■ INTERMITTENT EXPLOSIVE DISORDER

Psychological disorder causing violent behavior. Intermittent explosive disorder is an impulse disorder characterized by violent outbursts. These outbursts can be directed at others, property, or one's self. It is unclear exactly how many people suffer from IED, and some experts believe that IED is nothing more than a by-product of other disorders. Researchers who study IED focus on brain functioning to learn about some of the potential causes of the disorder. Medication and behavioral therapies have been shown to help treat IED.

IMPULSE CONTROL DISORDERS AND INTERMITTENT EXPLOSIVE DISORDER

According to the authors of a 2006 article in the *European Psychiatry and Clinical Neuroscience,* impulse-control disorders can be characterized by both "repetitive behaviors and the inability to control these behaviors." They state that the criteria for such behaviors include a failure to resist an impulse that can harm others or oneself. Further, before engaging in the behavior, the person feels an increased level of tension or arousal. This feeling is released once the act has been committed. To put it another way, a person has an urge to do something and engages in the behavior to satisfy that urge.

Intermittent explosive disorder (IED) is an impulse-control disorder and has several characteristics. First, it is characterized by episodes of aggressive behavior. The outburst is considered to be out of proportion to the event that caused the anger. These outbursts occur repeatedly over time. According to the Mayo Clinic, the eruptions typically last between 10 and 20 minutes. People with IED often state that they feel the following when they are about to act out: chest tightness, tingling, tremors, and head pressure.

Another criteria for IED is the aggression cannot be explained by another disorder (physical or psychological). Men are more likely than women to develop intermittent explosive disorder, and most people with IED are relatively young—between late adolescence and late twenties.

Fact Or Fiction?

Drivers with road rage have intermittent explosive disorder.

The Facts: There is not enough research to definitively connect IED and road rage. In one study that appeared in 2002 in *Behaviour Research and Therapy,* the authors examined aggressive drivers with and without IED. They found very few differences between the two groups. Aggressive drivers with IED had slightly higher levels of impatience, hostility, resentment, and anger. However, the differences were not significant. The authors also found that aggressive drivers, regardless of whether or not they were diagnosed with IED, were significantly more hostile, assaultive, suspicious, and anxious than nonaggressive drivers.

It is unclear how many people in the United States have intermittent explosive disorder. The author of a 2006 study in the *Archives of General Psychiatry* estimates that 5.4 percent of the general population has IED. The author indicates that this figure increases to 7.3 percent if IED is measured using broader criteria.

A study published in a 2008 issue of the *American Journal of Orthopsychiatry* focused on the prevalence of IED in a Latino population. The authors found that 5.8 percent of those in the study could be classified as having IED in their lifetime. When looking at the prevalence of IED during the past year, only 4.1 percent of Latinos met the criteria. The authors also found that IED co-occurred with other psychiatric disorders, such as anxiety, depression, and conduct disorders. The frequent co-occurrence of IED with other disorders has led the authors to wonder if IED is a unique disorder or a common symptom of other psychological disorders.

In another study, published in a 2005 issue of the *Journal of Clinical Psychiatry,* the authors surveyed patients at an outpatient psychiatric facility. More than 6 percent (6.3) were classified as having a diagnosis of IED at some point in their lives. Only 3.1 percent were considered to currently suffer from IED.

A 2008 article in the *Bulletin of Clinical Psychopharmacology* also presents information on the prevalence of intermittent explosive disorder. The authors of this article looked at the prevalence of IED among patients in an inpatient psychiatric unit within a university hospital. They discovered that 37.9 percent of patients had some form of an impulse-control disorder. Among all patients, 14.6 percent were diagnosed with IED.

Authors of a 2008 study in *Aggressive Behavior* examined the differences among people with intermittent explosive disorder, people who engaged in verbal aggression, and a third group of people with a personality disorder not connected to IED or verbal aggression. The authors compared people diagnosed with IED to people without IED but who engaged in verbal aggression against others. The only reason the second group was not classified as having IED is their lack of physical aggression. However, they met the verbal aggression component of an IED diagnosis.

There were some similarities between the groups. Both had similar scores on self-reported aggression and anger measures. Both groups also had a moderate to severe level of psychosocial impairment. This means the psychological problems associated with IED and with verbal aggression caused people to have difficulties functioning in social and work settings. However, people diagnosed with IED had more aggressive personalities than those who only engaged in verbal aggression. Those with IED were also more impulsive and showed emotional lability. Emotional lability is a condition in which a person's mood rapidly changes, and emotional reactions are out of proportion to events

IED AND INJURING ONESELF

Authors of a 2008 study in *Psychiatry Research* examined how often people with IED engaged in aggression against themselves. The

DID YOU KNOW?

Student Suicide Trends in the United States

Sex and Grade Level	1991	1993	1995	1997	1999	2001	2003	2005	2007
				Percent of students who seriously considered suicide[1]					
Total	29.0	24.1	24.1	20.5	19.3	19.0	16.9	16.9	14.5
Male									
Total	20.8	18.8	18.3	15.1	13.7	14.2	12.8	1 2.0	10.3
9th grade	17.6	17.7	18.2	16.1	11.9	14.7	11.9	12.2	10.8
10th grade	19.5	18.0	16.7	14.5	13.7	13.8	13.2	11.9	9.3
11th grade	25.3	20.6	21.7	16.6	13.7	14.1	12.9	11.9	10.7
12th grade	20.7	18.3	16.3	13.5	15.6	13.7	13.2	11.6	10.2
Female									
Total	37.2	29.6	30.4	27.1	24.9	23.6	21.3	2 1.8	18.7
9th grade	40.3	30.9	34.4	28.9	24.4	26.2	22.2	23.9	19.0
10th grade	39.7	31.6	32.8	30.0	30.1	24.1	23.8	23.0	22.0
11th grade	38.4	28.9	31.1	26.2	23.0	23.6	20.0	21.6	16.3
12th grade	30.7	27.3	23.9	23.6	21.2	18.9	18.0	18.0	16.7

(continues)

DID YOU KNOW? (CONTINUED)

Percent of students who attempted suicide[1]

Total	7.3	8.6	8.7	7.7	8.3	8.8	8.5	8.4	6.9
Male									
Total	3.9	5.0	5.6	4.5	5.7	6.2	5.4	6.0	4.6
9th grade	4.5	5.8	6.8	6.3	6.1	8.2	5.8	6.8	5.3
10th grade	3.3	5.9	5.4	3.8	6.2	6.7	5.5	7.6	4.9
11th grade	4.1	3.4	5.8	4.4	4.8	4.9	4.6	4.5	3.7
12th grade	3.8	4.5	4.7	3.7	5.4	4.4	5.2	4.3	4.2
Female									
Total	10.7	12.5	11.9	11.6	10.9	11.2	11.5	10.8	9.3
9th grade	13.8	14.4	14.9	15.1	14.0	13.2	14.7	14.1	10.5
10th grade	12.2	13.1	15.1	14.3	14.8	12.2	12.7	10.8	11.2
11th grade	8.7	13.6	11.4	11.3	7.5	11.5	10.0	11.0	7.8
12th grade	7.8	9.1	6.6	6.2	5.8	6.5	6.9	6.5	6.5

[1] Response is for 12 months preceding the survey.

The percent of students who have seriously considered suicide declined between 1991 and 2007. However, the percent of male students who attempted suicide increased, while there was a slight decrease of female students attempting suicide. People with IED sometimes attempt suicide.

Source: *Health, United States, 2008.* Centers for Disease Control and Prevention, 2008.

authors discovered that 12.5 percent of the subjects with IED had attempted suicide. Another 7.4 percent had engaged in self-injurious behavior. However, the authors also found that those who engaged in self-injurious behavior also experienced major depressive disorder, post-traumatic stress disorder, and a dependence on drugs. It is difficult to say whether the behavior is strictly a result of IED, other factors, or a combination of IED plus other factors.

CAUSES OF INTERMITTENT EXPLOSIVE DISORDER

In order to better understand intermittent explosive disorder, researchers have focused on how the brain functions. In particular, they look at the parts of the brain that influence emotions, impulses, decision making, and various cognitive functions. In a 2007 study in *Biological Psychiatry,* researchers reported findings on brain functioning in people with IED. They found that the amygdala in the brain was overactive in IED subjects when they were shown pictures of people with angry faces. The amygdala is a part of the brain that helps with the processing of fear and anger. If the amygdala is not working properly, a person can react too strongly when they experience stimuli (events, people, places, and so on) that can produce fear or anger.

The authors also found there was no overactivity of the amygdala when IED patients were shown pictures of other facial expressions. This is important because it may help explain why people with IED overreact to events that are considered "threatening" and not to other events. These findings provide some evidence of the biological nature of IED—a faulty amygdala in the brain can help contribute to someone's explosive anger in situations where it is not warranted.

A 2002 article in the *Proceedings of the National Academy of Sciences* provides support for the idea that people with intermittent explosive disorder have impaired executive functions. Executive functioning refers to cognitive abilities such as problem solving, judgment, planning, decision making, the inhibiting of inappropriate behavior, and social conduct. It makes sense that a person's executive functioning is impaired if he or she has IED. Impulsive behavior results, in part, because of the person lacks the ability to inhibit the abnormal behavior.

The authors of the 2002 article had people with IED and a control group perform cognitive-ability tests. They found that those with IED had impaired cognitive functions. For example, those with IED performed worse on a facial recognition test. This is a test where first pictures of facial expressions are shown, then the people being tested have to identify the expressions. Those with IED made more errors when trying to judge expressions of anger, disgust, and surprise than those people in the control group. This means that people with IED have trouble identifying the reactions or emotions of others when they are angry, disgusted, or surprised. In turn, a person with IED may react inappropriately, such as having a violent outburst.

Chemicals in the brain, known as **neurotransmitters,** also have an influence on impulsive behavior. This was demonstrated in a study published in a 2009 issue of *Psychopharmacology.* The authors of this study examined whether a neurotransmitter influenced self-injurious behavior in people diagnosed with intermittent explosive disorder. Reduced levels of the neurotransmitter **serotonin** have been connected with aggression. The authors of this study had people with and without IED drink a mixture that temporarily lowered serotonin levels. Others in the study were given a placebo, or unmedicated mixture, so the authors could have a comparison group. There were two key findings. First, people who received the drink mixture were willing to inflict more harm on themselves compared to those who drank the placebo. Self-harm was measured by the intensity of a shock the person would self-administer if she or he failed to complete a task before someone else. This means that people who drank the mixture gave themselves stronger shocks when they failed to win at a task, compared to those who only had the placebo drink.

Second, regardless of whether a person received the drink mixture or a placebo, subjects who were diagnosed with IED gave themselves stronger shocks, compared to those without IED. Taken together, these findings show that low serotonin levels are connected with self-injurious behavior. Individuals with IED have been shown to have lower serotonin levels compared to those without IED. People diagnosed with IED are at an increased risk of hurting themselves because of their impulsive-aggressive nature.

TREATING INTERMITTENT EXPLOSIVE DISORDER

As with other psychiatric disorders, intermittent explosive disorder can be treated with medications and psychological therapy. Referring back to the 2006 study in the *European Archives of Psychiatry and Clinical Neuroscience,* the authors report that both divalproex and lithium have been shown to help reduce impulsive aggression. Other medications that have been effective include carbamazepine, phenytoin, fluoxetine (an antidepressant), and propranolol (a beta blocker).

Very few studies have examined how well psychological therapies work on intermittent explosive disorder. One study, according to a 2008 article in the *Journal of Counseling and Clinical Psychology,* reports on the effectiveness of cognitive behavioral therapy for treating IED. The authors found that cognitive behavioral therapies were effective in helping treat IED; in particular, aggressive behavior diminished. The ability of people with IED to better control their anger improved, with this improvement lasting beyond the treatment phase. Based on the results of this study, the authors believe that the executive functioning ability of people with intermittent explosive disorder may be impaired.

See also: Anger Management; Road Rage; Violent Behavior, Causes of

FURTHER READING

DiGuseppe, Raymond, and Raymond Chip Tafrate. *Understanding Anger Disorders.* New York: Oxford University Press, 2006.

Libal, Autumn. *Drug Therapy and Impulse Control Disorders.* Broomall, Pa.: Mason Crest Publishers, 2007.

■ LEGAL INTERVENTIONS

The involvement of the law—usually by the actions of law enforcement agents—in the course of arresting or attempting to arrest lawbreakers, suppress disturbances, maintain order, or other legal actions.

The 2006 report of the Department of Justice (DOJ) found that 856,396 people serve as local police officers, with 105,933 additional officers serving at the state level. Federal agencies have another 156,607 people. Including the courts and prison systems, the Bureau of Justice Statistics reported that some 2.3 million people worked in the criminal justice system in 2003. That represented an 81 percent rise in manpower since 1982.

What do all those law enforcement people do? Traditionally, police worked to deter crime by patrolling the streets (usually in police cars) and apprehending offenders. Since the late 1960s, the police in many communities have been emphasizing crime prevention through **community policing.** Community policing is a partnership between police and the citizens of a community to prevent crime. Responsibility for reducing crime is placed on local police commanders who work with residents to identify threats to the community.

A 1995 National Institute of Justice report discusses some community policing strategies. Departments set up neighborhood-based offices or stations and designate "community" or "neighborhood" officers. Foot patrols are used to help an officer get to know the neighborhood and its residents even as the officer's presence discourages criminal activity. Some police departments also use bicycle patrols and involve residents in local community patrols and citizen police academies.

Police agencies that responded to the 1995 DOJ report listed a number of benefits of community policing. These benefits included a physical improvement in neighborhoods and more positive attitudes toward the police among residents. Police officers or deputies felt greater satisfaction with their job and the crime rate in localities using community policing dropped.

How does the typical police officer see his or her job? In a 1995 article in the *City Journal,* George L. Kelling, a social scientist specializing in police matters, discussed an internal survey of the New York Police Department. Kelling found that 91 percent of the officers believed that the public had little understanding of police problems. In addition, 75 percent disagreed with the statement that police officers and the public had a good relationship, while 81 percent agreed with the statement that the public believed police used too much force.

Kelling also offered an interesting view of the problems of policing from an officer's point of view. Seeing a heated argument between a cab driver and passenger, an officer has three hypothetical responses. By intervening before things get violent, the officer keeps the peace but gets no official recognition. By waiting until the argument escalates, the officer could make an arrest and receive official credit. If, however, the officer intervenes and something goes wrong, the result could be a complaint that affects the officer's future career.

POLICE ABUSE

One of the biggest challenges for police in the United States is building and maintaining positive relationships with their community. The vast majority of police officers are positive role models in their communities, enforcing the law fairly and justly. However, since the beginning of law enforcement efforts more than 200 years ago, there have been conflicts between officers and citizens. A notable example took place in 1999. In February, Amadou Diallo, a Nigerian immigrant, was killed by New York City police officers who fired 41 shots at the unarmed man. That June, Chicago police shot and killed two African Americans, LaTanya Haggerty and Robert Russ, at two traffic stops, six hours apart. Perhaps the best-known case took place in 1991. After a car chase, Los Angeles police officers repeatedly struck Rodney King with a nightstick. The beating changed the way many citizens viewed police behavior, in part because the incident was videotaped. The video was shown nationwide for weeks and triggered riots in Los Angeles that resulted in a billion dollars' worth of damage.

Fact Or Fiction?

The police come down hard on people depending on their race or where they come from.

The Facts: A 2002 study in the journal *Criminology* covered 3,000 police encounters in two cities. Rather than race, citizen behavior was the most significant factor in triggering disrespectful policing. People with low self-control, males, young people, and those with low-income levels tended to receive more disrespect from police. The study found that people from minority groups actually showed less disrespect for the police than whites. However, the study also revealed that police did display a cultural bias against those they perceived to be on the social and economic fringes of society.

In 1996, just five years after the Rodney King case, another video of Los Angeles police officers beating an immigrant man and woman after a lengthy car chase received national attention. In 2000 a series of abuses in Los Angeles once again brought the practices of the LAPD to the nation's attention.

In a 2002 article in the *Journal of Criminal Justice,* incidents of police misconduct were related to public opinion. The most significant drops in approval ratings followed the Rodney King video. The number of people expressing confidence in the police dropped by 43 percent in the white community, 49 percent in the Hispanic community and by 50 percent in the black community. On a positive note, all drops in confidence were eventually erased and levels of confidence returned to normal with the passage of time after each incident.

More than 75 percent of minority residents felt the behavior described above was not an exception but regular behavior by officers on the force. Research reported in a 2000 issue of the *Journal of Criminal Justice* points out that citizen complaints are most commonly related to how well the people in the police match the people in the community. Age also becomes a factor. Police departments with older officers tend, on average, to have more citizen complaints made against them.

Residents were so outraged by the treatment they were receiving from the police that the Los Angeles Police Department (LAPD) made significant changes in its procedures to address the problem. The city appointed a new police chief, who made efforts to hire officers from various ethnic backgrounds so that the profile of the police force more closely matched the profile in the community. The city also set up a civilian review board, a group of citizens to deal with cases of possible police misconduct. Although the new board addressed many community concerns regarding police behavior, it also faced many challenges, specifically resistance from officers over decisions being made by people outside the force. The city also set up an independent team of investigators to examine reports of poor behavior by the police. In the past, internal members of the police force would look into such charges.

Efforts such as those completed by the LAPD can be done in any community and within any police force. Each is an attempt to improve relationships between local residents and the police. When relationships are strong, citizens can play an active role actually assisting police in the battle to reduce violence in their neighborhoods.

CITIZEN DISRESPECT

While Los Angeles has received much attention for some of the challenges they have faced, the issue confronting most police departments is a lack of respect for police officers. People expect the police to protect them and their property. Unfortunately, when confronted by police, some people fight back or verbally abuse officers.

Civilians may have reasons for resisting the efforts of local officers. A 2003 article in the *Journal of Criminal Justice* points out that one major cause for resistance is a belief that the officer is acting unjustly. If many officers gather around a person, he or she may feel threatened, overwhelmed, and scared. If the police stop a driver in a high traffic location or many bystanders are watching, embarrassment may trigger some defiance of the police in an effort to save face or preserve social standing in the community. The feeling of having one's freedom restricted, real or perceived, may also trigger resistance. Not surprisingly however, the best predictor of whether individuals will resist police efforts is whether or not they were using alcohol or drugs at the time of arrest. These substances lower inhibitions, leaving people likely to act in ways they would not even consider when not under the influence of a drug.

A 2001 study on police use of force by the International Association of Police Chiefs found that between 1995 and 2000, 46 percent of the traffic stops in which police had to use force occurred when the subject was under the influence of alcohol or drugs. Intoxicated drivers were three times more likely to attempt force against police, most often using their automobiles, knives, or baseball bats.

Police work can be dangerous, and some officers have engaged in misconduct. However, the overwhelming majority of police officers dedicate themselves to controlling violence and making sure citizens are safe.

Q & A

Question: How can I help local police make my community safer?

Answer: You might consider some of the community involvement programs run by police departments. D.A.R.E., or Drug Abuse Resistance Education, teams police officers and teachers to discuss drug problems and also involves parents. G.R.E.A.T., Gang Resistance Education And Training, is a joint outreach program of the Federal Bureau of Alcohol, Tobacco, and Firearms and local police departments to schools, students, and parents. The Law Enforcement Explorers offers a more hands-on experience with police work for 14- to 20-year-olds. This program is a joint effort between police and the Boy Scouts. You can also discuss other community involvement programs such as Block Watch and citizen patrols with your family members. Inquire about any of these programs with your local police force. If the programs aren't available, you may be able to encourage local police to start some of them.

See also: Communities and Violence; Criminals and Violent Activity; Drugs and Violence; Social Costs of Violence

FURTHER READING

Asirvathan, Sandy. *Police and Policing.* Philadelphia, Pa.: Chelsea House Publishers, 2002.

Dunham, Roger D., and Geoffrey P. Alpert. *Critical Issues in Policing: Contemporary Readings.* Long Grove, Ill.: Waveland Press, 2004.

■ MEDIA AND VIOLENCE

The means of communication that reach large numbers of people, including newspapers, magazines, radio, television, films, and electronic communication. In bringing information and entertainment to millions of Americans, the media also depict many acts of violence. In the news media, consumers encounter wars, terrorist attacks, and a variety of crimes. In the entertainment media, many of the adventure and suspense stories that people read, see on the screen, or interact with in computer games contain violence. Even the music industry has developed a cult of violence, with songs about crime, shootings, police confrontations, and the mistreatment of women.

Violence in the media is not new. The first black-and-white film was a cowboy movie about a train robbery. Both the outlaws and the sheriff's posse blazed away with their six-shooters, and people fell dead. What is different today is the nature of the violence. It is more graphic, more sexual, and more frequent. But does it inspire acts of violence?

HOW MUCH VIOLENCE IS THERE?

When it comes to television, the most comprehensive research on violence was released in 1998. Responding to a challenge from a U.S. senator, the cable television industry paid for a three-year study involving researchers from four universities. In each year, the researchers studied 2,700 programs from 2,000 hours of broadcasts on 20 channels. They found that 61 percent of the shows contained violent content and that very few shows established consequences for the perpetrators. According to the Nielsen Group, which rates TV-show viewership, children watch 20 or more hours of television per week on average. Based on that estimate, children see approximately 10,000 acts of violence every year, mostly by characters who show no feelings about their actions and who, for the most part, go unpunished.

In "Carmegeddon," a game cited in a 1999 article in *Time* magazine, players could run over as many as 330,000 people going through all the levels in the game. Imagine how many more acts of aggression we view today.

Q & A

Question: If I watch a murder mystery at the theater, am I just going to snap one day and recreate what I saw?

Answer: Acting violently comes from a combination of many factors, both personal and environmental. However, for some people the interaction with media violence can cause a problem. In the lead-up to the massacre at Columbine High School in 1999, one of the two gunmen put up a customized version of the shoot-'em-up game "Doom" on his Internet Web site. The game featured two shooters, and all of the people being shot were unable to fire back. The pair also made a videotape for a class project in which they roamed the school, shooting athletes. In this case, the relationship between fantasy, media, and actual commission of a crime yielded 13 murders and the suicides of the two young gunmen.

WHAT IS THE EFFECT?

While researchers have managed to count violent episodes in the media, they have not been as successful in measuring the impact of that violence—especially on young people. Some scientists have dismissed laboratory experiments that measure aggressive reactions to violence in the media as having no relation to real life. Even when researchers agree that violence does have an effect, they disagree as to what that effect may be.

A 2001 article in the *Journal of the American Academy of Child and Adolescent Psychiatry* summarized research in the field from the previous 10 years. According to the article, people who view many hours of violence on television are more likely to exhibit violence as a means of solving conflict than those who watch less TV. The younger children are, and the more violence they are exposed to, the more aggressive their behavior and their scores on psychological tests.

A 2006 article in the *Annual Review of Public Health* reviewed the research on media violence and violent behavior. The authors state the research is clear that short-term exposure to media violence stimulates people to act in aggressive and violent ways. The authors go on to state that long-term exposure leads people to change the way they think and view violence, making it more acceptable in everyday life.

Most of the research also identifies yet another issue, the desensitization of individuals to violent acts. In other words, the more violence a person is exposed to, the less likely that person is to be shocked, appalled, or angry about violence in his or her neighborhood. People who see violence come to accept it and are less likely to try to reduce violence.

In her book *The Loss of the Assumptive World,* grief therapist Linda Goldman discussed the impact of media on the way young people see the future. The "assumptive world" is a reflection of what kids take for granted: safety, love, trust, self-worth. As children view more and more violence, it erodes their idea of how safe they, or the world around them, may be. Goldman noted that children who survive terrible events feel unsafe, less valued, and more vulnerable. She believes that children who see no future for themselves experience hopelessness and fear. They are also more likely to turn to negative behaviors.

In the 2001 *Report from the Surgeon General on Youth Violence,* the country's highest-ranking public health officer discussed the impact of violence in the media. Electronic media can be found in almost every household and young Americans spend more than four hours a day with television, computers, VCRs and DVDs, and a variety of video games. Psychologists currently believe that some of the new interactive media may influence children's behavior even more powerfully than earlier products. In other words, the act of killing someone in a video game may make more of an impression than passively watching a killing on a TV screen.

Testing such beliefs, however, will not be possible until psychologists and other social scientists develop more accurate ways of measuring exposure to violence and how the patterns of that exposure vary depending on age, gender, and other distinctions.

A DISTORTED IMAGE

When violence in movies and television becomes part of the political debate in the United States, the focus is almost always on its impact on children. In his 2003 book *The 11 Myths of Media Violence,* media professor W. James Potter argued that the emphasis on young people is misguided. Exposure to violence affects all ages, all ethnicities, and both genders. By focusing on just one group, he maintains, the nation will not resolve the larger issue. Managing the amount of violence to which people of all ages are exposed is a better approach.

One of the myths that Potter addresses is the common belief that media violence is merely a reflection of violence in society. Potter used the research on the National Television Violence Study, which reviewed programming 17 hours each day on 23 channels and found approximately 18,000 acts of violence every three weeks, the equivalent of 936,000 acts of violence per year. Considering the fact that there are many more channels than the ones monitored, and seven more hours to the day, Potter estimated that television shows about

2.5 million violent acts each year. Using government crime statistics, he found that 1.4 million violent offenses were actually committed in the United States during the previous year. Is television a reflection of the real world? Potter says it is not. In his opinion, television grossly overestimates the degree of violence in American society.

A study described in a 2003 article in the *Journal of Criminal Justice and Popular Culture* monitored the crimes portrayed in the three highest-rated criminal justice dramas. Murder or attempted murder made up 66 percent of the offenses, with property crimes like theft or fraud making up only 9 percent of these prime-time crimes. Consulting the Federal Bureau of Investigation's Uniform Crime Reports for the same year, researchers found that in New York (the setting for two of the programs), most of the crimes were against property, with violent crime making up only 26.4 percent of the total and murder less than 1 percent. In Boston, the locale of the other show, violent crimes made up only 21 percent of crime total, with murder coming in at 0.4 percent.

Admittedly, a murder probably makes for a more suspenseful episode than a car theft. A sensational murder will also capture more news attention than an interfaith gathering to pray for peace. These choices, however, do not reflect reality. They serve more as advertisements for a violent, hostile world—and motivate some people to react more aggressively than the real world needs.

Fact Or Fiction?

One person can do very little about violence on TV.

The Facts: Dealing with violence on television may need the work of many people, but it can begin with one person. A good starting point is to examine the way you watch TV. Another is by learning how to examine and criticize programs. Acquiring media literacy skills is an important step in controlling TV rather than having TV control you.

Read and research the problems associated with TV violence. What are the financial and organizational reasons for violent shows and films? Look for ways to bring up the problem in schoolwork, such as essays or reports. Discuss this issue with your teachers and with local TV stations. Most stations these days have Web sites. Why not contact them and express your concerns?

You might even help to bring your school and a local TV station together on a project, like videotaping public service announcements about violence. There's a lot to be done—and a lot one person can do to make a difference.

See also: Communities and Violence; Criminals and Violent Activity; Gang Violence; School Violence; Violent Behavior, Causes of

FURTHER READING
Edgar, Kathleen J. *Everything You Need to Know about Media Violence.* New York: Rosen Publishing Group, 1998.
Kirsh, Steven J. *Children, Adolescents, and Media Violence.* Thousand Oaks, Calif.: Sage Publications, 2006.

■ RAPE
See: Sexual Violence

■ REHABILITATION AND TREATMENT OF PERPETRATORS
Efforts to help those convicted of crimes return to and function effectively in society. Originally, prison sentences were intended solely as punishments. However, officials in the correctional system have long believed that one of their missions is to rehabilitate offenders.

Conviction for a particularly violent or other serious crime can put a person in prison for life. However, the overwhelming majority of prisoners serve shorter terms. If, upon release, they can become productive citizens, not only they but also society benefits.

Some former prisoners return to criminal behaviors. Repeating or returning to criminal behavior is called **recidivism.** Corrections experts measure recidivism rates to determine the success or failure of rehabilitation efforts.

INFLUENCES ON RECIDIVISM
In 2002, the Bureau of Justice Statistics released the results of a study of 272,111 former prisoners over a three-year period after their release. That number represented about two-thirds of the prisoners released from state prisons that year. The bureau requested records from 15 states with large and diverse populations. Of the released prisoners,

60 percent were rearrested and 40 percent were reconvicted within three years of leaving prison. The Kentucky Corrections Division has reported similar numbers: 40 percent of violent offenders were back in jail within one year of release. The division also reported that 33 percent of weapons violators and 14 percent of sex offenders were also back in prison within a year of release. Offenders do not necessarily return to prison for the same crime that resulted in their earlier conviction. Many were sent back for technical violations such as using alcohol or drugs, failing to report for curfews, or not attending treatment meetings.

While people commonly believe crime involves large amounts of money, studies contradict this notion. A 2000 article in *Criminology* suggests that crime is a lot of work, with street criminals engaging in robbery, burglary, and theft, auto theft, con games, forgery, and drug dealing. While some criminals take in thousands of dollars a month, 50 percent would be described as low-earning, and 63 percent would be described as inefficient, having to commit a large number of crimes, which increases the chances of arrest. A 2003 study in the *American Journal of Sociology* found criminals "earning" thousands of dollars a month but also losing money to expensive drug addictions and from being incarcerated. Released inmates with a criminal record often face difficulty in getting jobs. Also, a 2003 research paper for the Urban Institute's roundtable on prisoner reentry to society and work found a 30 to 50 percent unemployment rate among newly released prisoners, and an earnings rate of only $250–$500 a month.

Psychological problems may also affect a released inmate's chances of being sent back to prison. A 2002 study in the *Journal of Interpersonal Violence* of previously convicted adolescents found that those who had difficulty in controlling their behaviors, especially impulsive behavior, often were arrested again. A 2001 study reported in the *International Journal of Offender Therapy and Comparative Criminology* followed 480 graduates, ages 15 to 40, of a correctional "boot camp" (a prison that uses military-style training) for three years. Researchers found that the earlier in life individuals commit violent offenses, the more difficulty they have fitting into society and the more likely they are to commit crimes as they grow older.

A number of programs try to help rehabilitate those who have been convicted of violent crimes. Many prisons have treatment programs for inmates. After their release, many former prisoners participate in parole and community service.

TREATMENT PROGRAMS
IN DETENTION AND PRISON

After an individual's conviction for a crime, he or she is sentenced to prison. That sentence can offer that individual an opportunity to change. Prison authorities try to encourage and guide that change through prison-based treatment programs. A wide variety of approaches have been tried over the years, but research has indicated which are most effective. A 2001 study on European methods published in *Psychology in Spain* and a 2002 study by American researchers in *Behavior Science and the Law* reached similar conclusions. Programs that teach inmates how to control their behavior and improve their attitudes prove the most effective in reducing recidivism.

A 2006 study in the journal *Psychology of Addictive Behaviors* reports on the effectiveness of a meditation program used in a prison setting. The authors found that inmates who went through the 10-day meditation program had better results after being released from prison. In particular, they showed significant decreases in the use of crack, alcohol, and marijuana. The authors also reported better psychosocial outcomes for these inmates.

Behavior modification is a form of treatment that uses psychological tools such as positive and negative reinforcement (rewards and punishments) to promote changes in behavior. Prison behavior modification programs try to teach appropriate responses to conflict. Instead of getting angry and punching someone, offenders learn to react more appropriately.

One system of positive reinforcement is based on a **token economy**, an arrangement in which those who act in an appropriate way receive tokens that can be used to purchase desirable items. This system works best in controlled environments. A token to get a snack has little value when one can walk to the nearest convenience store and buy snack foods. It becomes more desirable in a setting in which one is not free to move about. Prison is the ultimate controlled environment, where token economies have been at work since the 1970s. The technique is considered especially useful in dealing with young offenders. A 2002 report, *What Works in Reducing Young People's Involvement in Crime*, by the Australian Institute of Criminology, confirms this system's usefulness.

Cognitive–behavioral treatment is a form of therapy that helps people understand and control the thoughts and emotions that cause various behaviors. In prison-based programs, inmates usually work in groups rather than individually to learn positive social skills.

DID YOU KNOW?

National Rate of Recidivism, Within Three Years, of State Prisoners Released in 1994, by Prisoner Characteristics

Prisoner charact- eristics	Percent of all released prisoners	Rearrested	Reconvicted	Returned to prison with a new prison sentence	Returned to prison with or without a new prison sentence
All released prisoners	100	67.5	46.9	25.4	51.8
Gender					
Male	91.3	68.4	47.6	26.2	53.0
Female	8.7	57.6	39.9	17.3	39.4
Race					
White	50.4	62.7	43.3	22.6	49.9
Black	48.5	72.9	51.1	28.5	54.2
Other	1.1	55.2	34.2	13.3	49.5
Ethnicity					
Hispanic	24.5	64.6	43.9	24.7	51.9
Non-Hispanic	75.5	71.4	50.7	26.8	57.3
Age at release					
17 or younger	0.3	82.1	55.7	38.6	56.6
18–24	21.0	75.4	52.0	30.2	52.0
25–29	22.8	70.5	50.1	26.9	52.5
30–34	22.7	68.8	48.8	25.9	54.8
35–39	16.2	66.2	46.3	24.0	52.0
40–44	9.4	58.4	38.0	18.3	50.0
45 or older	7.6	45.3	29.7	16.9	40.9
Number of released prisoners with information	272,111	183,674	127,620	64,116	140,953

Source: Bureau of Justice Statistics, 2002.

They learn to solve problems instead of acting aggressively, positive reasoning instead of hair-trigger reactions, and thoughtful responses instead of aggressive behavior. Prisoners can acquire many different strategies for dealing with conflict in a positive fashion rather than resorting to violence as a solution.

Cognitive-behavioral therapy concentrates on a series of mental steps—thoughts and emotions—that occur in the brain before taking an action. By breaking the **cycle of events,** as it is called, professionals can help inmates keep an action from taking place. The process is called **relapse prevention.** In a 2000 article in *Behavioral Science and the Law,* describing a relapse-prevention program for violent sex offenders, the author points out that no single event triggers relapses to violent behavior. The crime proceeds from a series of emotions, fantasies, and thoughts to a plan not only for an attack but also to remove inhibitions against committing the attack. By the time a person has stifled the feeling that "I shouldn't be doing this," nothing will stop the resulting violence. Cutting off the thought and emotional process earlier can prevent the criminal act. The goal is for offenders to learn to take responsibility for their actions, recognize when they are moving toward violent behavior, and to control the impulse.

PAROLE AND COMMUNITY SERVICE

Parole is an agreement between a prisoner and prison authorities. The prison agrees to release the prisoner as long as he or she agrees to be supervised and follow a set of rules or conditions. The purpose of these conditions is to keep the released prisoner from returning to prison. The Texas Youth Commission, for example, has established programs for young offenders that include education, therapy while in the correctional system, work programs, and training designed to increase self-discipline. The Texas program has reduced recidivism for youth who participate in the program compared to young prisoners who chose not to take part.

According to the Bureau of Justice Statistics, in 2006 approximately 40 percent of parolees were returned to prison because they were rearrested or violated the conditions of their parole. This figure has remained relatively consistent since 1990.

Community service describes efforts to improve a community or neighborhood. Courts can impose community service in addition to a prison sentence or as an alternative to prison. Sometimes offenders are set to work menial tasks, such as cleaning up parks or roadsides. Often, however, community service involves helping victims of crimes similar to those the offender committed, or educating the public about the behavior that led to the offender's arrest. A 2000 report on the Ohio community service program appeared in *Corrections Management Quarterly*. The article stated that participants in the community service program had a recidivism rate of only 20 percent, compared to a 36 percent rate for the general prison population. In addition, the more hours of community service prisoners performed, the less likely they seem to be to commit new crimes.

TEENS SPEAK

I Didn't Realize How It Hurt

Jake is a freshman in a junior college. He volunteers in several local programs.

"I used to think the scariest thing I had ever had to deal with was standing in front of a judge and admitting I beat up my girlfriend—at least she used to be my girlfriend. That's over. We got into an argument over my looking at another girl, and I popped her—right as a cop came around the corner.

"I thought I got off pretty lightly in court, just a small fine and 250 hours of community service. Then I found out they'd assigned me to the local women's shelter. I worked at the front desk, helping to admit women and their children to a safe place where they could get away from abusive relationships."

Jake shudders. "At first, I almost wished they had put me away. Now I understand why they did it. What I saw at the shelter really scared me. Some women came in covered with blood; others were just so scared that all they could do was cry for hours. I saw one woman come in seeming just fine. She didn't look beat up, she wore nice clothes; you'd think she could be anyone's mom. For a while I couldn't figure out why she was there. Then her boyfriend turned up yelling. He began throwing chairs around, finally breaking a window. The guy was crazy."

He shrugs. "My community service is over now, but I go over to the Teen Center and talk with the guys there. I tell them that abuse lasts longer than the 10 seconds it takes to hit someone. It can stay with people for life. It's not the most comfortable thing, having people stare at you while you talk about your far-from-proudest moments. But I know a lot of these guys, and hopefully they can learn something to keep them from ending up where I did."

Rehabilitating people who have broken the law, especially violent offenders, is not a simple task, nor is it accomplished easily. If people can be saved from a life of crime, however, the task must be attempted—if only to avoid adding to the already crowded prison population in the United States.

See also: Criminals and Violent Activity; Sexual Violence; Violent Behavior, Causes of

FURTHER READING
Blue, Rose, and Corinne J. Nader. *Punishment and Rehabilitation.* Philadelphia, Pa.: Chelsea Press, 2001.

■ REVENGE, CYCLE OF

Violence creating more violence. The cycle of violence often refers to two phenomena. Violence that provokes someone to seek revenge is one form of the cycle of violence. Revenge is emotion-driven violence. The victim has been injured and angered. The angrier the victim is, the more likely it is that she or he will retaliate. This in turn leads the other person to seek revenge, and the cycle continues.

The cycle of violence also refers to intergenerational violence, when violence is transmitted from parents to children. Research shows that children who are exposed to **domestic violence,** or who are physically, sexually, or psychologically abused by family members, are at much greater odds of repeating the behavior when they are adults.

REVENGE AND RETALIATION AS A MOTIVATION

What motivates revenge and even violent retaliation? According to the authors of a 2009 article in *The Arts in Psychotherapy,* revenge is defined as "retaliation in response to a perceived injustice against a person (or a group with whom that person feels identified)." Revenge can be a strong motive to commit an act of violence against another person.

In another 2009 article, in *Organizational Behavior and Human Decision Processes,* the author examined how offender motives can influence revenge. The author learned that victims' perceptions of why someone committed an offense influences the desire to seek revenge. In particular, if a victim believes an offender acted out of malice or greed, then retaliation will more likely be considered instead of other coping strategies. The author mentions that anger plays a key role in this process. The perceived severity of the offense, combined with feelings of anger, contribute to the likelihood of seeking revenge. The more severe the offense and the greater the anger, the more likely revenge will be sought.

In a 2007 article that appeared in *Social Justice Research,* the authors discuss the many emotions that might motivate someone to seek revenge. By reviewing the works of others, the authors believe that the key emotion that motivates revenge is anger. In particular, it is the intensity of the anger that can lead a person to retaliate against others.

There are questions as to how someone can overcome any personal objections to hurting another person. According to the authors of a 2007 article in the *Journal of Experimental Social Psychology,* one way to overcome this is by engaging in "moral justification." This happens when a person believes a harmful behavior is justified because it serves a righteous or valued social purpose. In other words, the person believes that violence is justified because of the greater good it will cause.

According to the authors of a 2007 article in the *Journal of Pediatric Psychology,* retaliation is often motivated by a person's desire to restore or maintain an image, or reputation, after an incident with someone else. The authors examined attitudes about retaliation among African-American adolescents who had been assaulted. The majority of these adolescents believed it was acceptable to hit a person if that person had just hit you. However, the children in this study did not believe that revenge is good. Although this seems contradictory, the authors believe that it may indicate that the children believe in self-defense but not necessarily in retaliation. The authors also discovered that adolescents were more likely to endorse retaliation if they believed their parents were supportive of fighting. In fact,

DID YOU KNOW?

Gang Violence in Los Angeles, February 2009

	Crime Category	This Month	Feb. 2008	YTD	Last YTD	% of Change
1	Homicide	11	10	24	26	7.7
2	Aggravated Assault (Excl. ADW on PO)	177	277	391	448	-12.7
3	Attacks on Police Officers (Agg. & Simple)	3	8	10	8	25.0
4	Rape	1	4	6	6	0.0
5	Robbery Excl. Carjacking	138	204	350	407	-14.0
6	Carjacking	3	6	13	17	-23.5
7	Kidnap	2	8	9	7	28.6
8	Shots Inhabited Dwelling	20	7	39	23	69.6
9	Arson	0	0	1	*N.C.	3.2
10	Criminal Threats	39	67	119	139	-14.4
11	Extortion	1	4	2	4	-50.0
	TOTAL	395	545	964	1085	- 11.2

*N.C.=Not Calculable

Gang-related crimes are often driven by a cycle of revenge. In one month alone, there were 395 violent actions by gang members who were known to the Los Angeles Police Department.

Source: *Citywide Gang Crime Summary.* Los Angeles Police Department, February, 2009.

the parents' actual attitudes were not as important as the perceived attitudes by the adolescents.

In another article, in the *Journal of Family Issues* in 2008, the authors focus on gender differences in the acceptance of retaliatory violence. First, the authors found that men are more likely than women to approve the use of violence. That is no surprise, as decades of research have consistently shown this to be a fact. However, men and women equally disapprove of men using violence against women, even if women acted violently first. This finding was stronger when the target was a spouse compared to a female acquaintance. The authors note that women are partially protected by social norms, as violence against women is generally discouraged.

A 2002 report commissioned by the U.S. Secret Service and the U.S. Department of Education highlights just how dangerous revenge can be in motivating violence. *The Final Report and Findings of the Safe School Initiative* reviewed 37 acts of targeted school violence that involved weapons. The incidents occurred between 1974 and 2000. According to the authors of the report, 61 percent of the offenders were motivated by revenge.

The authors of a 2008 study in the journal *Basic and Applied Social Psychology* looked at the issue of whether retaliation is in proportion to the original offense or exceeds the original offense. They found that people who sought revenge inflicted harm that seemed out of proportion to the original offense. As a result, the offender then saw himself as a victim. The authors also discovered that those seeking revenge were satisfied when they felt the revenge was fair.

In a 2008 article in the *Journal of Personality and Social Psychology*, the authors examined the emotional consequences of revenge. They conducted an experiment to see how people would feel if they punished someone for acting inappropriately. The authors reported that people believe they will feel better by punishing a person for bad behavior. What was discovered is that people actually felt worse after inflicting a punishment. People who were not given an opportunity to punish an offender actually felt better than those who had the opportunity and used it. This study indicates that exacting revenge on someone does not necessarily mean that the victim will feel better.

Q & A

Question: Do nations use the threat of revenge to prevent other nations from attacking them?

Answer: Throughout history, nations have vowed to defend themselves if attacked. Today, the same holds true, although it can be more complicated because of international politics. The United Nations (UN), headquartered in New York City, is an international organization designed to promote peace and cooperation among the nations of the world. Despite this organization, however, countries continue to threaten other countries with aggression and retaliation.

The best example comes from the United States and former Soviet Union (USSR). During the period in history known as the cold war, each country developed thousands of nuclear missiles, capable of destroying the world. Because the United States and USSR were enemies, they vowed to destroy one another if ever attacked. This produced the doctrine of mutually assured destruction. If one country launched a nuclear missile against the other, missiles would be launched in turn against the aggressor. Because the missiles contained nuclear warheads, the United States and Soviet Union would destroy each other. According to Greenpeace International, the United States has approximately 9,962 nuclear weapons, while Russia has 16,000 nuclear weapons. This is more than enough weapons to ensure one country will not attack the other.

A similar study appeared in a 2007 issue of the *Journal of Social and Personal Relationships*. The authors examined emotions and revenge, and the results of the research support the belief that anger is a critical emotion in motivating someone to seek revenge against another person. However, those who had sought revenge often experienced remorse after the act. Instead of the revenge making a person feel better, the person often felt worse. In addition to feeling bad about the act, the findings also showed that people would often be fearful of further retaliation.

INTERGENERATIONAL TRANSMISSION OF VIOLENCE

The cycle of revenge also refers to intergenerational violence. In this case, children learn from their parents about the acceptability of violence. When the children become adults, they are much more likely also to use violence. If the violent adults have children, their children will be exposed to violence and believe it is acceptable. This is how the cycle continues.

In a 2007 article that appeared in the *Journal of Family Violence*, the authors looked at intergenerational violence. As expected, it was found that adults who were abused as children were more likely to abuse their own children. Witnessing violence as a child increased the odds of engaging in domestic violence as well. The authors also discovered that the more exposure to violence a child witnessed, the more often that child engaged in domestic violence as an adult. This indicates that the use of violence is, at least in part, a learned behavior.

Authors of a 2009 study in the *Journal of Youth and Adolescence* discovered something different when examining intergenerational violence. Some of the findings were typical. Adolescents who were exposed to domestic violence were more likely to engage in violence and delinquency during their adolescent years. It was also discovered that exposure to severe domestic violence as an adolescent helped predict engaging in partner violence as an adult. However, being abused as a child did not predict engaging in partner violence as an adult. This finding contradicts other research that has shown being abused as a child influences the likelihood of engaging in violence as an adult.

Another study, which appeared in a 2006 issue of *Child Abuse & Neglect,* also reported such findings. The authors of this study found that if a child was exposed to family violence or physically or sexually abused, the risk of that child engaging in domestic violence as an adult increased by 200 to 300 percent. However, there was no connection between being abused as a child and engaging in child abuse as an adult.

A 2009 article in the *Journal of Criminal Justice* examined intergenerational violence among men who batter their partners or spouses. The authors found a relationship between being physically maltreated as a child and committing intimate partner violence as an adult. However, there was no relationship between witnessing parental violence and engaging in similar violence as an adult. The authors also found that children who received corporal punishment by their mothers were less likely to engage in intimate partner violence. This finding complicates our understanding of intergenerational violence: Violence by a father may contribute to the problem, while violence by a mother may help inhibit the problem.

See also: Family Violence

FURTHER READING

Hardy, Kenneth V., and Tracey A. Laszloffy. *Teens Who Hurt: Clinical Interventions to Break the Cycle of Adolescent Violence.* New York: Guilford Press, 2006.

Minow, Martha, and Nancy L. Rosenblum. *Breaking the Cycles of Hatred: Memory, Law, and Repair.* Princeton, N.J.: Princeton University Press, 2003.

■ ROAD RAGE

Violence shown by drivers in traffic, often as a sign of stress. Practical demonstrations of road rage can be found on almost any major roadway. Imagine a beautiful, sunny day with you and your friends out on a short cruise. The goal is to have fun and enjoy the day. Then, a car buzzes your front bumper while changing lanes, almost knocking you and your friends into a ditch. Or someone is driving 45 miles per hour in the left lane of the highway. She refuses to move out of the lane to allow you to pass. How do you react?

Most people might express some annoyance or laugh it off. For too many drivers, however, the highway has become something like the Wild West, a place where any inconsiderate or clumsy driving requires revenge or punishment with hair-trigger aggression. According to a 2001 article in *Social Psychiatry and Psychiatric Epidemiology,* the term *road rage* did not exist until the media began using it in the 1980s. The researchers in the article found that over 50 percent of all drivers have experienced a road rage incident in the last five years.

DEGREES OF ROAD RAGE

A 1999 study in the *Chronicle of the American Driver and Traffic Safety Education Association* noted four degrees of road rage. The first degree involves a gesture or a few select words directed at the offending driver. In the second degree of rage, an exchange of gestures or cursing occurs between the parties involved. This exchange may escalate into expressions of anger that distract both drivers from surrounding traffic, increasing the chance of a crash.

As the level of aggression builds to the third degree, drivers begin harassing actions such as flashing high beams, impeding the progress of other vehicles or, when being tailgated, stopping quickly to frighten other drivers. Reaching the fourth and greatest degree of rage, drivers become still more aggressive, having verbal or physical confrontations with the people who offended them, causing injury. Drivers may also display weapons as threats while cursing people who are driving too slowly. In some situations, the weapons even get used. Researchers view this fourth degree as the most dangerous scenario—one that has occurred with increasing frequency over the past 10 years.

In 1997 testimony before Congress, the administrator of the National Highway Traffic Safety Administration reported that aggressive driving contributed to one-third of automobile crashes nationwide in the previous year—and two-thirds of the 41,907 crash-related deaths.

No clear-cut, single reason can explain why people allow their anger to control how they drive. However, researchers have developed a few explanations.

SELF-DETERMINATION THEORY

In 2001, researchers at the University of Houston used what they called the **self-determination theory** to explain aggressive behavior on the road. This theory is based on the idea that free will can be used to understand people's motivations and personalities and tries to categorize people into two personality types. **Autonomy-oriented** types believe that they determine their own responses and actions. **Control-oriented** types are more likely to attribute their behaviors to the actions of others. To put the difference simply, the first type represents students who do homework because they see a benefit in doing well in class or earning good test scores, or they enjoy learning something new. The second type would include students who do their homework only because their parents make them do it.

Autonomy-oriented people generally have a more positive self-esteem, are more likely to take responsibility for their actions, and are less likely to become angry when provoked. Control-oriented people are more likely to react based on the pressures of the world around them and attribute their behavior to those forces rather than to their own actions.

How does this theory relate to driving? The University of Houston researchers found that control-oriented drivers showed more aggression on the road and were more likely to show anger, get into accidents, and receive tickets for poor driving. They also reacted more aggressively to hostile gestures, slow or rude drivers, traffic delays due to road construction, and the presence of police.

A 2001 study published in the *Social Science Journal* found that although many drivers responded with road rage when traffic slowed, reckless driving by others was more likely to initiate a confrontation. The researchers discovered that differences in age or gender did not change their findings. Drivers decided whether to retaliate solely based on how angry they were about the triggering incident.

THE VIEW FROM BEHIND THE WHEEL

If you drive, you probably know whether you get angry while you are on the road. If you do, you must consider the possible consequences of your actions. Aggressive drivers get more tickets, become involved in more accidents, and place those in their vehicles at greater risk. In the long run, consequences may include higher insurance costs and the possibility of hurting another person—possibly someone you care for. The way you react is not controlled by the actions of others. If you get cut off in traffic, you may be annoyed, but it is not a personal attack.

Experts suggest that you slow down if you are angry. Speed plays a significant role in crashes. You can choose the driving speed for your car, regardless of the way others might be driving. Imagine you need to drive across town. It's a 10-mile drive and the speed limit is 45 miles per hour. Driving at the speed limit, you will arrive in a little over 13 minutes. If you decide you are in a hurry and take off at 55 miles per hour, you will arrive in just under 11 minutes. How important is that two minutes, especially when driving 10 miles over the speed limit increases your changes for a ticket, or a crash in which you and others may be injured?

If you find that you have a tendency toward road rage, practice stress management. When you feel yourself getting angry, take deep breaths, count to 10, play music you enjoy, whatever it takes to stay calm. In the long run, you win, because if you can learn to manage your emotions when you drive, you can use those skills in other aspects of your life as well.

Drivers have complained about increasing aggressiveness on the nation's highways for years. Uncontrolled road rage can lead to dangerous situations not only for the targets of angry motorists but also for the innocent drivers around them. People get into plenty of trouble by swinging baseball bats or pipes at people who provoke them. Turning a ton and a half of glass and metal—one's car—into a weapon can have serious, even fatal, consequences.

See also: Fight or Flight Response; Violent Behavior, Causes of

FURTHER READING

Eberle, Paul. *Terror on the Highway: Rage on America's Roads.* Amherst, N.Y.: Prometheus Books, 2006.

Winters, Adam. *Everything You Need to Know About Being a Teen Driver.* New York: Rosen Publishing Group, 2000.

■ ROBBERY
See: Social Costs of Violence

■ SCHOOL VIOLENCE
Any behavior that violates a school's educational mission, spoils a climate of respect, or jeopardizes the intent of the school to be free of aggression against persons or property, drugs, weapons, disruptions, and disorder. Based on this definition provided by the Center for the Prevention of School Violence and one offered by the Federal Bureau of Investigation (FBI), school violence can include anything from bullying to homicide.

THE SCOPE OF THE PROBLEM
Throughout the 1990s, school violence was associated with a series of sensational news headlines. In 1995, a 17-year-old in Giles County, Tennessee, brought a .22 rifle into his school, killing a teacher and a classmate. In Paducah, Kentucky, in 1997, a 14-year-old brought a pistol, two rifles, two shotguns, and 700 rounds of ammunition to school. Three girls died, and five other students were wounded. In 1998, an 11-year-old and a 13-year-old set themselves up as snipers outside their middle school in Jonesboro, Arkansas. After setting off a fire alarm, they opened fire as schoolmates filed into the parking lot. Four students and a teacher died.

In 1999, the most sensational incident to date took place. Two boys, 17 and 18 years old, brought guns and bombs into Columbine High School in Littleton, Colorado. They killed 12 students and one teacher and took their own lives. In 2005, a 16-year-old shot and killed nine people, including his grandfather and students and teachers at a high school in Red Lake, Minnesota.

A 2000 Secret Service report summarized 37 school attacks since 1974, attacks which left 54 dead and 124 wounded. Described as "an epidemic of school violence," these incidents triggered an avalanche of research, policy statements, and programs to address the issue of violence within the school setting.

The Centers for Disease Control and Prevention (CDC) collects information from teens across the nation by asking a series of questions. This annual study, the Youth Risk Behavior Surveillance System (YRBSS), revealed the following in a 2010 report:

- In a survey of high school students, more than one-third of respondents reported being in a physical fight in the previous 12 months. Of those, 3.8 percent were injured seriously enough to require medical treatment by a doctor or nurse.

- About 5.6 percent of students carried a weapon such as a gun, knife, or club on school property within the month before the survey.

- Five percent of students did not go to school on one or more of the past 30 days because they felt unsafe at school or on their way to or from school.

- Nearly 7.7 percent of students had been threatened or injured with a weapon on school property one or more times during the past 12 months.

THE CONTAGIOUS NATURE OF SCHOOL VIOLENCE

When people describe the increase of school violence as an "epidemic," they do not refer to a disease carried by germs but a phenomenon that spreads through psychological means. Although personal decisions play a part, participants in a 1998 Department of Justice research forum pointed out that violence can become "contagious." Violence can reach epidemic proportions when young people decide to carry weapons and act more aggressively, causing others around them to do the same.

The media can also play a major part in spreading the infection. Researchers became aware of this effect decades ago. A 1986 article in the *New England Journal of Medicine* linked media coverage of suicides with sudden surges in teen suicide rates. A similar connection exists between media coverage and school rampages. In the weeks after the exhaustively covered tragedy at Columbine High School, every state except Vermont reported threats of similar actions. Would-be copycats were discovered planning gun attacks or bombings in high schools and middle schools as far from Littleton, Colorado, as California and Florida.

In 2001, a pair of high school boys in Kansas were caught before they attempted an imitation of the Columbine massacre. That same year, officials were unable to stop a 15-year-old boy in Santee, California. His attack resulted in the murder of two students and the wounding of 13 others.

Admittedly, screaming headlines and top story status on newscasts help to focus attention on a problem. The saying in newsrooms across the country is short and brutal—"If it bleeds, it leads." In the case of school violence, however, such coverage also serves to promote additional violence, in the opinion of some media observers.

FEAR OF CLASSMATES

In his book *School Violence*, Jeff Jones quotes President Bill Clinton as saying, "In most schools it's not the sensational acts of violence, but the smaller acts of aggression, threats, scuffles, and constant back talk that take a terrible toll on the atmosphere of learning, on the morals of the teachers, on the attitudes of students."

Fear is the enemy of education. Students and teachers are unable to concentrate if they are continually looking over their shoulders. Unfortunately, at too many schools in the United States, that is exactly what they are doing.

In 2003, the Departments of Justice and Education issued a joint report, "Indicators of School Crime and Safety." Among the many facts and figures in the report was a statistic on the percentage of students between the ages of 12 to 18 who feared an attack at school or on the way to or from school. In 1995, that figure stood at 12 percent of students. In 1999, the figure dropped to 7 percent, in 2001 to 6 percent, and in 2005, it was also at 6 percent.

The data from the study showed that students have good reason to be fearful in their school environment. There were an estimated 1.5 million nonfatal victimizations at school in 2005. The data show that 14 percent of high school students (grades 9–12) reported being in a fight on school grounds. Twenty-eight percent indicated they had been bullied, with 9 percent saying they had been shoved, tripped, or spit on. Of those who were bullied, 24 percent were injured. From July 1, 2005 through June 30, 2006, there were 14 students killed while at school. Although this number is extremely low given the millions of students in school, it is still high enough to make students fearful of the same thing happening to them.

TEENS SPEAK

A Deadly Lesson

Steve is a high school senior and the quarterback on his school's football team.

Steve recalls Brian, a fellow student. "'Brian Brain-dead,' we used to call him—that, or 'Stick-boy' because he was so skinny. Those were the nicer names we used, ever since he transferred to our school last year. Brian never objected to the names or the pranks people pulled on him. Either that, or he quickly learned not to.

"I suppose we shouldn't have been surprised at his interest in school shootings. Everybody knew that would be his report for Contemporary Studies. I should have said something when one of the guys on the team tore up Brian's charts. But it was Brian Brain-dead, so who cared? Ralph was a linebacker—he could have broken Stick-boy over one knee."

Steve shakes his head. "Brian went home during lunch. I thought he was getting replacement charts. Instead, he came back with his dad's gun.

When he walked to the front of the class and shot out the window, I thought, 'I'm dead.' I mean, I was everything he hated—one of the popular kids, an athlete on the football team.

Then we heard the sirens in the distance. From the look on his face, Brian suddenly realized that being locked up in Juvie would be 10 times worse than school. So he used the gun—on himself."

Steve shuts his eyes. "Afterward, the news people were all over us. They wanted to know what movies Brian watched, what computer games he played—what they could blame. Nobody wanted to listen when we said we were all to blame. When I saw that gun, I kept thinking, 'I'm getting just what I deserve.' Too bad there's no way I can make it up to Brian."

SCHOOL-BASED PREVENTION STRATEGIES

Educators across the nation recognize the destructive nature of violence on the school environment. As a result, administrators have increased their efforts to keep the school environment positive and learning-oriented. Some schools have assigned staff or volunteers to monitor bathrooms and hallways and routinely check bags, desks, or lockers. Other administrators have brought uniformed police officers into their schools and utilized metal detectors and surveillance cameras. These efforts are aimed at making the school environment safer and less violent so that students can focus on schoolwork rather than their safety.

Many schools have also established programs to teach students how to avoid violent situations and to keep conflicts from becoming violent. The following sections examine some of these initiatives.

Self-control

One of the core concepts behind any attempt to curb school violence involves teaching young people to manage or regulate their emotions. When people feel angry, they do not automatically have to act on that emotion. They can instead work through their problems instead of turning to violence. Unfortunately, many young people have been exposed to so much anger and violence that they have never developed the ability to control their emotions.

In 2000, researchers from the University of Southern California examined how exposure to violence may affect the way people manage emotions. Their findings suggest that children who witness violent behavior are more likely to see violence as an acceptable response to conflict. Children who are victims of violence, not just witnesses, also have difficulty managing their emotions.

The Michigan Model for School Health Education identifies three steps to managing anger. First, individuals must identify what their triggers are. A **trigger** is an event that stimulates anger. When people know which events are most likely to make them angry, they can either avoid those situations or prepare themselves to deal with the tension. Knowing what is coming makes the situation less likely to get out of control.

Second, individuals need to recognize their anger. Anger is a natural emotion. People need to understand how their bodies respond to feelings of anger. How does the body respond to a trigger? How does the anger build?

The third step involves finding ways to cool the anger. Some people learn to remove themselves from environments that make them angry. The most effective approaches separate an individual from a conflict. Talking with someone about the problem can help, as can exercising or participating in an activity that one enjoys, like reading or even taking a nap.

Negotiation

Negotiation is a method of resolving conflict between two people—or groups—by conferring until a mutual agreement is reached. Suppose you lend money to a friend on several occasions. The amount is adding up, and you want him or her to pay you back. Your friend might respond, "I can't give you that much—I don't have it." By negotiating, you may be able to work out a system of repayments.

Sometimes people disagree on what is appropriate. By sitting down and discussing the issue, they may resolve the problem in such a way that everyone involved is satisfied with the result.

Mediation

One of the more popular approaches to curbing violence in schools is through **peer mediation,** a process by which a fellow student or member of the community helps resolve a conflict. A mediator is not just any student, however. He or she has received training in a six-step procedure:

1. Mediators explain that the arguing parties must reach their own agreement. In doing so, all sides need to respect one another, and allow one another to offer his or her case without interruptions.

2. Mediators ask each party to explain the problem and to express his or her feelings without becoming aggressive.

3. Each of the opposing parties is given time to state the problem.

4. Mediators restate and sum up the dispute based on what they heard and what they know about the problem. They may also ask questions to clarify the situation.

5. Mediators ask each side to come up with a solution for the problem and then restate their suggestions. Mediators do not offer their own solutions.

6. When both sides reach an agreement, they sign a contract that sets out what each party is willing to do.

A mediator's job is to look objectively at a conflict, not show favoritism, and come to an appropriate resolution.

Communication skills

Effective communication involves not only being able to say what one feels but also being able to hear what others have to say. Saying what one feels requires an ability to express oneself in a positive way. Describing

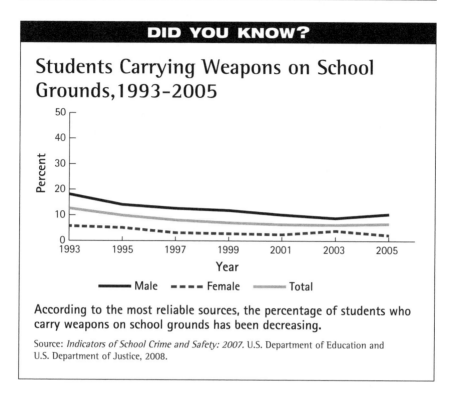

DID YOU KNOW?

Students Carrying Weapons on School Grounds, 1993–2005

According to the most reliable sources, the percentage of students who carry weapons on school grounds has been decreasing.

Source: *Indicators of School Crime and Safety: 2007.* U.S. Department of Education and U.S. Department of Justice, 2008.

what one is thinking or feeling without hurting someone else is a skill that does not come naturally to many people. It takes practice.

Situations in which people try to express why their feelings were hurt or how they have been offended are often tense. No one wants to say something that may end a friendship or start an argument. However, if one doesn't speak up, then acts that cause hurt feelings or cause offense will continue, which can cause even more damage to a friendship or relationship.

Communication requires not only speaking but also listening. Learning that one's words or actions have hurt someone's feelings can be difficult to hear. It is all too easy to be defensive. Then, while one plans how to respond to criticism, he or she stops listening. One cannot plan a counterattack and really listen to a complaint at the same time. The person who thinks ahead to how he or she should respond will probably miss the most important part of the discussion: *why* a friend is hurt or offended.

By keeping one's emotions in check and really paying attention to what a friend is saying, a person will have a much better understanding of the situation and will be able to come to a more effective solution to the conflict.

Programs to resolve conflict among students can play an important role in improving conditions in not only school but also their community. Those skills can make a positive difference in one's relationships. They can also help prevent school violence. While reports of school violence have decreased in recent years, the problem still remains a troubling one for too many students in the United States.

See also: Assault and Bullying; Criminals and Violent Activity; Media and Violence; Teens and Violence; Violent Behavior, Causes of

FURTHER READING

Orr, Tamra. *Violence in Our Schools.* New York: Franklin Watts, 2003.

Thomas, R. Murray. *Violence in America's Schools: Understanding, Prevention, and Response.* Westport, Conn.: Praeger Publishers, 2006.

■ SELF-MUTILATION

A deliberate but nonlethal injury to the body, including activities such as cutting or scratching oneself, burning, hitting oneself hard enough to bruise the skin or break a bone, or hair pulling. Even persistent nail-biting can be considered a low-level form of self-mutilation. The condition is also known as self-harm or self-injurious behavior. Whichever the name, it describes a serious and complicated disorder—one that is difficult to overcome.

WHY WOULD PEOPLE HURT THEMSELVES?

Pain is something everyone has to deal with. Athletes know the "agony of defeat"—especially the special pain of making a mistake on the playing field. Maybe someone just ended a relationship that he or she thought would last a lifetime. Talking to parents, teachers, or friends may help to relieve the pain. In time, most painful episodes pass and life moves on. Unfortunately, life does not move on for everyone, and for some the stress and guilt associated with a painful episode is turned inward. A small but growing percentage of people choose to inflict external physical damage on themselves as a way of coping with internal pain.

In his book *Living on the Razor's Edge,* family therapist Matthew Selekman discusses some of the factors that push young people into behaviors like "cutting." Cutting is just what it sounds like, using a razor or other sharp instrument to make cuts on the body. Selekman points out that the act of causing the injury is an attempt to relieve a significant emotional pain. It is also a sign that an adolescent needs assistance in working through an emotional crisis. Young people who practice this behavior may not have an underlying personality disorder and should not automatically be considered a victim of sexual abuse or someone with suicidal tendencies.

Psychologists and physicians have learned that causing bodily harm to oneself is usually a way of coping with feelings of unworthiness and a lack of connection to parents and other adult figures. What Selekman calls a **family breakdown** may cause some adolescents to feel as though their parents do not even know they exist. Feelings of unworthiness or abandonment are large burdens to carry, and adolescents who injure themselves are doing so to deflect some of their emotional pain. The key for these youths is to find out what is missing and try to rebuild that relationship.

A second reason for self-mutilation can be found in the pace of life today. Classes, organized sports, after-school jobs and activities can be stressful. The pressure to achieve academically and personally can be overwhelming. In the absence of a positive way of coping with such strains, some young people turn to self-injuring behaviors.

Third, Selekman points out that our society's demands for a quick resolution to problems may lead to incomplete treatment. Many young people who injure themselves are placed on medication, treating the symptom and hiding the fact that deeper emotion-based issues may be at the core of the problem rather than chemical imbalances in the brain.

In 2002, researchers for the American Psychological Association tried to identify ways of providing positive and negative reinforcement for young people who exhibit self-injuring behaviors. **Positive reinforcement** can be described as a reward or desirable result obtained from a behavior. It encourages repetition of an action. In contrast, **negative reinforcement** is a punishment or undesirable outcome obtained from a behavior. It discourages repetition. Most parents react with concern and attention when their children hurt themselves. Children who believe they are not noticed may learn that by hurting themselves, they receive the attention they desperately wish for.

Positive reinforcement may also come from peers, leading young people to take up or keep practicing the behavior. If friends think that cutting is cool, they may convince others to do so as well. If friends respond positively, giving people the attention they want, that reinforces the behavior.

Q & A

Question: How can I tell if one of my friends has a problem with self-mutilation?

Answer: It won't be easy, mainly because people try to hide this behavior as best as they can. However, scars or sores that your friend has explained away as cat scratches may be warning signs, especially if these injuries appear on the forearms.

Burn marks that appear to be caused by a cigarette or a flame may also be a sign of self-hurting. If your friend's explanation is brief, and he or she seems to be avoiding any discussion of his or her injuries, these too may be signs. None of these signs offer proof beyond a doubt. All of them can be caused by other things, and often are. If you know your friend is hurting emotionally, being aware of his or her pain and providing support may be a first step in helping him or her move away from self-injury.

TREATMENT OPTIONS

An important aspect in helping friends or family members to stop injuring themselves is to alter the way they think about themselves. Consider this common scenario: A mother expresses anger at her teenager, prompting thoughts such as "I'll never be good enough," and then self-abusive behavior begins. The place to intervene is at the middle step. It is impossible to control what a parent says or does, but one can control one's own responses to their words and actions. Individuals who cut or burn themselves feel poorly about themselves. Changing how one reacts to criticism and learning to recognize one's personal strengths can lead to a more positive result.

Because stress is such a significant factor in self-injury, learning techniques to manage stress can help. Exercise, meditation, keeping a journal, and many other techniques can help to improve one's outlook on life and move away from damaging behavior.

People struggling to stop self-injuring behaviors face a range of treatment options, depending on the amount of repetition and the severity of danger. In less severe cases, individuals may be able to find strategies for helping themselves by readings books on the subject. In more severe cases, medication, psychological therapy, or partial or inpatient hospitalization may be necessary.

Whatever form of treatment is needed, those who cut or engage in other forms of self-harm need help. Self-mutilation is an especially saddening form of violence because people direct it against themselves.

See also: Suicide

FURTHER READING

Clark, Jerusha. *Inside a Cutter's Mind: Understanding and Helping Those Who Self-Injure.* Colorado Springs, Colo.: NavPress, 2007.

Winkler, Kathleen. *Cutting and Self-mutilation: When Teens Injure Themselves.* Berkeley Heights, N.J.: Enslow, 2002.

■ SEXUAL VIOLENCE

Physical act of aggression that includes a sexual act or sexual purpose. The World Health Organization (WHO) defines sexual violence in *The World Report on Violence and Health* as "a sexual act, an attempt to obtain a sexual act, unwanted sexual comments or advances, or acts to traffic a person's sexuality, using coercion, threats of harm or physical force, by any person regardless of relationship to the victim, in any setting, including but not limited to home and work."

Q & A

Question: Isn't rape an issue that only involves women?

Answer: Rape is an issue important to everyone in a society. Expressing violence through sexual acts is wrong. Furthermore, while women make up the large majority of rape victims, men are also victims. The Bureau of Justice Statistics states that in 2007, 4.5 percent of surveyed inmates reported being sexually assaulted. Given the number of prisoners in the United States, this means approximately 70,000 inmates were sexually assaulted.

The victims include people of all ages and economic brackets–college students, young professionals, middle-aged people in wealthy suburbs, poor people in urban neighborhoods, even grandparents in nursing homes. Women, however, are overwhelmingly the targets of sexual violence. According to a Department of Justice report, the victims in 94 percent of completed rapes, 91 percent of attempted rapes, and 89 percent of both completed and attempted sexual assaults were women.

TEENS SPEAK

I Used to Be a Hero

Vince is large for his 17 years. He is presently suspended from his school's football team until a court hearing over accusations of rape.

"Not too long ago, people smiled when I walked by them in school. They cheered me on the football field, saying I would take the team to the state championships. That's all over now."

His shoulders hunch a little as he goes on. "A bunch of us were unwinding after a big game. Some beers, some music—a little company. I was with a cheerleader named Sherry—a really cute girl. We'd fooled around a little before . . . before what happened."

"This time, we really got into it, hot and heavy. And then she starts saying 'no.'"

Vince takes a deep breath. "Maybe if I hadn't been drinking—I don't know. I thought I could make her say 'yes.' Sherry was crying when I left."

"Nowadays when I walk down the halls in school, people look at me differently. And, of course, I'm off the team. College scouts were beginning to come around but not anymore."

He squeezes his eyes tightly shut. "All I ever wanted to do was play ball. But now, because I wanted somebody to say 'yes' instead of 'no,' I've sent my whole life down the tubes."

RAPE

The Federal Bureau of Investigation (FBI) runs the Uniform Crime Reporting service, which annually tabulates reports from law-enforcement agencies across the country. In 2002, according to those statistics, 95,136 forcible rapes were committed. However, not all rapes are reported. According to the Bureau of Justice Statistics, in 2006 there were approximately 192,320 attempted and completed rapes. An estimated 49.2 percent of rape victims reported the crime to the police. By comparison, only 25.7 percent of victims reported an attempted rape.

Who committed these offenses? When you hear the word *rape,* do you picture a stranger lurking in a dark alley? Or do you imagine a young man out on a date or a friend, even a relative? A 2002 report by the Department of Justice found that in 66 percent of sexual assault cases, the offender was someone the victim knew—a family member, a friend, or an acquaintance.

Defining rape

Forcible rape, as defined by the FBI's Uniform Crime Reporting system, is the carnal (sexual) knowledge of a female against her will.

Until the 1970s, U.S. laws defined rape as sexual penetration of a woman by a man who was not her husband, a crime under the English Common Law upon which American law is based. However, the Common Law was established through court cases dating back more than 700 years, much of it at a time when women were considered the property of their husbands who could force their wives to have sex if they desired. Common Law tended to protect men from accusations of rape rather than protecting women who suffered as a result of a rape.

Social changes, especially the rise of the feminist movement in the late 1960s, challenged this historical definition of rape. Increasingly, people in the United States and elsewhere viewed rape as a crime that has less to do with sex and more to do with violence and power.

Identifying possible rapists

In his book *Men Who Rape: The Psychology of the Offender,* A. Nicholas Groth, a clinical psychologist, identified four types of rapists. Federal and state law enforcement agencies use those categories to prevent rape and help capture perpetrators.

- The power-assertive rapist is usually aggressive, meeting his victims in settings like bars. He likes to control and degrade victims but does not intend to kill. His crimes are based on opportunity—he doesn't usually single out victims. Statistically, this type is responsible for approximately 40 percent of rapes.

- The power-reassurance rapist lacks the social skills to develop relationships with women and is often not athletic or aggressive. This type of rapist usually selects and stalks a victim. He may take trophies of his "conquests" or write about his activities in a diary. He often has a fantasy of a consensual relationship with a woman and is the least violent rapist. This type of rapist accounts for approximately 27.5 percent of rapes.

- The anger-retaliatory rapist feels hostile toward all women, has an explosive temper, and has little control over his impulses. He may also be a substance abuser. He does not single out a victim; his aggression is aimed at women in general. Attacks are usually spontaneous and brutal. Although he does not set out to kill victims, he may beat them to death if they resist or fail to escape. This type accounts for about 28 percent of rapes.

- The anger-excitation rapist enjoys torturing and killing victims for the thrill and sexual gratification of the acts. The person may select victims or take them in crimes of opportunity. This type of rapist is the most likely to kill and accounts for 4.5 percent of rapes.

Acquaintance rape

As the definition of rape has changed in society along with the legal interpretation, so has the image of the rapist. No longer is he seen as a stranger waiting in a dark corner. Today law enforcement officers and researchers recognize that a rapist could be a neighbor, a coworker, a friend of the family, a husband or boyfriend. A new term has evolved—**acquaintance rape**. It is a rape in which the victim knows the rapist. That category includes date rape—forced sex in which the perpetrator has an intimate or dating relationship with the victim.

Department of Justice statistics reveal that almost 70 percent of rape victims knew their assailant at the time of the incident. Although acquaintance rape is often portrayed as occurring on the first date, rape can occur at various stages of a relationship. Only one-third of date rapes take place on a first date. One of every four date rapes occurs after a couple has already dated a few times. Partners in long-term relationships commit an additional 30 percent of all acquaintance rapes.

Many Americans still believe a variety of myths about sexual relationships and rape. One myth is that a woman owes a man sex if he pays for the date. Another is that if a woman is sexually active, she does not really mean it when she say no; she's simply playing hard to get.

To avoid possible misunderstandings while dating, people must communicate about sexual behavior. Many men find it uncomfortable to bring up the subject, feeling it will "spoil the mood." Women may feel awkward saying something like, "I like you, and I'm having fun, but I do not intend to have sex tonight." However, a little embarrassment up front may save considerable trouble later.

Much of society still clings to these and other centuries-old myths, which place the blame on the victim. These myths about rape are not only untrue but may also be even illegal. In his book *Date Rape Prevention Book,* author Scott Lindquist points out a few of these myths:

- Victims must struggle for an attack to count as rape.
- If the victim has had sex before, he or she cannot bring a charge of rape against the perpetrator.
- Victims themselves are to blame if they allow a risky situation to develop.
- Women who dress provocatively should expect to be raped.

These beliefs are based on old legal doctrines that made it almost impossible to charge a rapist, much less prove the offense. They attempt to shift the responsibility for the offender's behavior to the victim and away from the rapist. Nothing could be more wrong. No rationale can excuse forced sexual activity.

Rape crisis centers

At a time when society offered little support for rape victims, a number of women in the 1970s founded rape crisis centers in their communities. Today most cities and towns have at least one such center. Many of them offer rape victims counseling and support groups. Victims also find advocates there willing to provide them with one-on-one support. For example, if a victim needs to go to a hospital for a medical examination, an advocate may accompany her to explain the procedures and provide assistance. If the victim decides to press charges against the rapist, advocates not only explain what to expect if the case goes to court but are often willing to stay with her throughout the trial. Advocates also provide help over the telephone on special lines open 24 hours a day, seven days a week. In addition, they try to keep the communities they serve informed about the problems associated with sexual assaults.

SEXUAL HARASSMENT

Sexual harassment is a form of sex discrimination that involves unwelcome sexual advances, requests for sexual favors, and other verbal or physical conduct of a sexual nature. Such harassment can create a hostile environment in the workplace or at school.

The law is vague in describing the specific acts that are considered harassment. In her book *Sexual Harassment, A Debate,* feminist philosopher Linda LeMoncheck points out that some forms of harassment are easily identified while others are based more on individual interpretation. One example is **sexual coercion,** the use of a supervisor's power to threaten an employee with being fired as a way of securing sexual favors. Sometimes, a supervisor may reward an employee who performs sexual acts with a promotion or a raise. This form of harassment is called **sexual bribery.** A supervisor who initiates physical contact—kissing, touching, pinching, or hugging—when that contact is not wanted is also easily identified as guilty of sexual harassment.

Sexual harassment becomes harder to identify (and prosecute) when the infractions are less obvious. If a female supervisor continues to ask an employee out on a date after he has already told her he is not interested, or a woman feels that a male colleague stares at her inappropriately, there is less agreement on whether a legal line has been crossed. Jokes that may be offensive to one woman but not offensive to her female coworkers are yet another example of the difficulties in drawing clear lines.

A key component to stopping harassing behavior early is communication. For instance, a woman can reduce the likelihood of harassment and establish what she believes to be appropriate behavior by being firm when she is offended. Speaking up and making sure your opinion is heard can go a long way in helping others to understand what you consider appropriate. If someone puts an arm around you as a form of greeting, and the act makes you uncomfortable, then a firm, "I'd prefer that you not put your arm around me," may take care of the problem. You have established a boundary. If the behavior reoccurs, then perhaps you should involve a teacher or the principal.

SEXUAL ABUSE IN COMMUNITY INSTITUTIONS

A 2002 article in the *Child Abuse Review* points out the growing number of scandals involving professionals who used their work to target and sexually abuse children in the course of the previous 15 years. Similar discoveries have been made in care for the aged. If, as A. Nicholas Groth and other psychologists have stated, sexual abuse is more about power than sex, it is not surprising that those who are least able to defend themselves are targeted.

Establishing firm statistics on the size of the problem of abuse in general and sexual abuse in particular is difficult. Shame and fear may keep many young victims from coming forward. These same feelings may keep elderly people silent as well. In addition, many people suffer from dementia—the loss of mental capacity—as they age. They may not be believed when they report abuse. Statistics cover only the number of abuse cases reported or the number of cases verified and these represent only the tip of the iceberg.

According to a 2006 report by The National Center on Elder Abuse, there were 191,908 substantiated claims of elder abuse in 2004. Of these verified claims, 1 percent were for sexual abuse. This means that there were 1,919 elder victims of sexual abuse in 2004.

A 2004 report to the British Parliament showed that 3 percent of calls to a national abuse hotline reported sexual mistreatment. It was the only growing category in the study. Interestingly, a suggested reason for the growth was that sexual predators who had previously focused on children now found themselves under heavier scrutiny and may have shifted their attention to a less-protected population.

The National Elder Law Network collects research on topics related to the elderly. Although the network has not been able to establish a single profile for abusers or their victims in elder abuse cases, it has established some common findings. Abusers tend to be nursing aides or orderlies who are experiencing burnout and have lost their sense of caring for the patients they serve. Facilities that have few staff to handle many patients are more likely to have cases of abuse. Abusers also tend to be young men with low levels of education and a lack of employment experience. In almost all cases, the victim is either mentally or physically unable to fight off an attacker or report the abuse. Only when a family member recognizes the abuse is it reported.

The Administration on Children, Youth and Families reports that in 2006, there were an estimated 3.3 million allegations of child abuse and neglect, involving 6 million children. Of these reports, in 28.6 percent of the cases, it was found that children were victims of abuse and neglect. In 8.8 percent of cases, a child had been sexually abused. A 2000 article in the publication *British Association of Social Workers* discussed the particular vulnerability of children to sexual abuse in institutional settings such as foster homes, clubs, schools, churches and synagogues, playgrounds, and family centers. In too many of these settings, sexual predators can establish themselves as caregivers or authority figures—coaches, teachers, religious leaders, or activity directors. By giving extra attention to children or promising candy, money, alcohol, or other enticements, they may lead children into an abusive situation.

Sexual violence is a difficult subject to understand in terms of the extent of the problem, the issues victims face, and even the importance of the crime. For example, the U.S. Supreme Court ruled against a law that established the death penalty for rapists on the grounds that victims survived the abuse. The question that remained unanswered was how the crime had impacted the lives of those survivors.

See also: Family Violence; Suicide

FURTHER READING

Bourke, Joanna. *Rape: Sexual, Violence, History (Reprint Edition).* Berkeley, Calif.: Counterpoint Press, 2009.

Feuereisen, Patti. *Invisible Girls: The Truth About Sexual Abuse—A Book for Teen Girls, Young Women, and Everyone Who Cares About Them.* Berkeley, Calif.: Seal Press, 2005.

Lindquist, S. *The Date Rape Prevention Book: The Essential Guide for Girls and Women.* Napierville, Ill.: Sourcebooks, Inc., 2000.

■ SOCIAL COSTS OF VIOLENCE

The price a society pays for crime and other violent behaviors. Some of that cost is financial, such as the loss people must deal with when thieves steal the family car or robbers make off with thousands of dollars from a bank or an armored truck. Taxpayers also pay; they finance efforts to prevent and punish crimes. Human costs are also associated with violence, including physical pain, mental suffering, and in some cases, loss of life.

The Centers for Disease Control and Prevention reports that in 2000, homicides and medically treated injuries resulted in costs of approximately $37 billion. Self-inflicted injuries accounted for another $33 billion. Cost estimates include medical treatment and lost wages.

Costs resulting from the commission of a crime can vary considerably depending on the source. Taking an average of the amounts lost in the 324,938 robberies reported in 2002, the Bureau of Justice Statistics report *Crime Victimization 2003* placed a value of $1,281 per robbery. Compare that to the $19,200 cost associated with a robbery in the 1993 book *Understanding and Preventing Violence*. According to this work, only 15 percent of the costs were financial—the monetary loss, society's loss of a worker's production, and emergency response to the crime. The rest represent nonmonetary losses including pain, suffering, risk of death, and psychological damage.

In its Web site on crime victims and civil justice, the National Center for Victims of Crime estimates that in 2004, crimes cost victims $345 billion.

ENFORCEMENT COSTS

Many of the costs of protecting a community are connected to its rate of violence. Essentially, as the rate of violence rises, so does the cost of police work. The Bureau of Justice Statistics counted 446,974 officers at the local level in 2004. In 2003, local governments spent a total of $57.5 billion on police. That money includes not only salary, but also the cost of training, operating facilities, non-officer support staff, automobiles, equipment, and general operation expenses. Based on the number of people in the United States, Americans spend approximately $286 per resident on local police. In addition, the report tabulated 200,000 law enforcement officers on the state level, and 93,000 federal agents authorized to make arrests.

The *Sourcebook of Criminal Justice Statistics 2005* issued by the Department of Justice looked at the figures differently. This report estimated the total expenditures for the justice system on the federal, state, and local level at more than $204 billion. Police protection accounted for less than half that figure (a little over $94 billion).

MEDICAL COSTS

The authors of a 2007 article in the *American Journal of Preventative Medicine* illustrate some of the medical costs associated with violent crime. Overall, approximately $4 billion were spent on medical expenses for violence-related injuries. The average medical costs associated with a nonfatal assault were $24,353. The average medical costs associated with nonfatal gunshot injuries were $15,293.

Violence that occurs between intimate partners cost almost $6 billion in 2003, according to the Centers for Disease Control and Prevention (CDC). Most of that cost, a little over $45 billion, went to direct medical care for victims of domestic violence. The remaining $2 billion was attributed to lost pay, lost production, and costs connected to the deaths of those who did not survive the violence.

PROSECUTION, INCARCERATION, AND REHABILITATION COSTS

In 2006, Department of Justice officials stated that expenditures for the criminal justice system exceeded $214 billion. Included in that number was spending by governments at various levels to provide police protection, operate and monitor correctional facilities, and fund judicial and legal activities.

The federal government spent about $36 billion on the criminal justice system, while state governments spent more than $69 billion, and local governments over $109 billion.

The costs of incarceration, or confinement in a jail or prison, are not as simple to determine as it might seem. On the federal level, corrections expenditures came to more than $5.5 billion. State prisons cost $39 million to run, while local governments spent $18 billion on jails.

According to a 2009 statement by the U.S. federal government, the average cost of incarcerating an inmate at a federal prison was $25,895 in 2008. There is a wide variation of costs across the 50 states. For example, in 2008 it cost California approximately $49,000 a year for each inmate. New Jersey estimated its yearly cost per inmate at $38,700. Other states, such as Virginia, have lower costs: between $20,000 and $25,000 per year for each inmate.

However, there are other costs that most people don't think about. Every benefit that a prisoner could potentially add to his or her community but cannot because of incarceration is considered a social cost. It includes the wages a prisoner might have earned if he or she was in society working and the value of what that prisoner might have produced on the job. The social costs also include the effects of incarceration on the prisoner's family, particularly on his or her children.

Fact Or Fiction?

Society doesn't owe criminals anything while they're in prison. They can sit and rot.

The Facts: While rotting in prison might punish an offender, that approach will hardly prepare an inmate for life after prison—or help to keep a former inmate from criminal activity that will guarantee a trip *back* to prison.

Providing rehabilitation services for people in prison serves both the inmate and the larger community. Helping prisoners develop skills to become productive members of society or learning a trade improve the prospects both for the inmate and the community.

A 2001 study of rehabilitation programs in the *Journal of Research on Crime and Delinquency* found that these efforts reduced the rate at which former prisoners returned to prison by 20 percent. Considering the vast prison population in the United States, imagine how many crimes rehabilitation may prevent.

Many prisons in communities across the United States have designed programs to help inmates overcome addictions or develop the skills necessary to remain free from crime. Some are self-help programs that assist prisoners in dealing with addiction or behavior problems. **Guided self-help programs** allow people to work on problems by themselves with information or advice from a therapist, a book, or a computer program.

Some prisons provide **group therapy**, a form of psychological treatment in which participants, with the help of a therapist, meet regularly to analyze their own and one another's problems. The interaction among the participants is an important part of the treatment process. **Individual self-help** allows inmates to deal with problems in their lives by learning to receive help, give help, and help themselves. Groups such as Alcoholics Anonymous have worked on the principle of individual self-help for years.

Many prisoners develop skills in communication, learning how to manage anger and avoid conflict. Some inmates even go out into the community to talk with young people about their experiences in prison. Kansas has a program that has seen the recidivism rate of inmates (the rate of people returning to prison after discharge) in such programs drop to one-half the national rate.

Q & A

Question: What factor has the largest effect on increasing the prison population?

Answer: According to the organization "Get the Facts," it cost the 50 states approximately $6.2 billion per year to imprison drug offenders in 2007.

Because alcohol and other forms of drug abuse are associated with many violent crimes, a number of prisons run programs for **drug rehabilitation,** a general term for programs and activities that help drug users overcome their addiction. According to the Office of National Drug Control Policy (ONDCP), 21 percent of all inmates in 1998 were drug offenders. An article appearing in the 2002 book *Treatment of Drug Offenders* pointed out that in-prison treatment centers are inexpensive compared to outpatient, community-based treatment. Reviewing three prison-based programs, researchers found that the cost per inmate ranged from $37 to $68 per week, while community treatment programs averaged over $600 per week. The ONDCP also emphasizes the importance of treatment, reporting that for every dollar spent on treating an inmate for addiction, the community benefits by three dollars, tripling the value of the treatment. These programs benefit communities by reducing the costs associated with crime and also by turning prison inmates into productive citizens.

The social costs of violence can be counted in billions of dollars and measured in the months of often painful medical treatment for survivors of violent crimes. Less easily measured is the fear that prevents people from attending an event that take place after dark or requires a trip through a dangerous neighborhood. The most painful statistic is the tens of thousands of people who pay the ultimate cost—losing their lives to violent crime.

TEENS SPEAK

Counting the Costs

Duane is 17, having spent the last four years as an inmate after being convicted of aggravated assault.

"I was 13 when a kid from school dissed me bad, and I beat him till he couldn't stand up. That got me four years."

He looks around the bare, institutional room. "So what did it cost? Time. Time with my family, as messed up as it is, it's still all I have. Time with my friends, my girl. They all forgot me. There isn't really a school here. The best I'll get is a General Education Degree (GED). My former friends are getting ready for college, and I'm here, falling farther behind.

"They have cars, I sit here. They have money, I sit here. They go wherever they want, and I freaking sit here." He smashes a fist into the thin mattress on his cot.

"You know what's weird? I'm scared to leave now. In here, I know the routine, I'm used to it. Out there, I have no life, and it scares me to have to start over.

"My advice? Listen to people. Sounds crazy, I know, but it would have made a difference. Listen when they tell you that what you think is cool really isn't. Listen when they warn you about people who will screw up your life. Listen when they tell you they love you, because you won't want to, and then they're gone. That's not cool."

See also: Alcohol and Violence; Criminals and Violent Activity; Drugs and Violence; Weapons of Violence

FURTHER READING

Harris Terrell, Ruth. *A Kid's Guide on How to Stop the Violence.* New York: Avon, 1992.

Libal, Autumn. *The Social, Monetary, and Moral Costs of Prisons.* Broomall, Pa.: Mason Crest Publishers, 2006.

■ SUICIDE

The intentional taking of one's own life. In 2005, the *Sourcebook of Criminal Justice Statistics* reported 12.7 suicides per 100,000 people in the United States. The rate was higher for those 80 years and older, with 18.7 deaths per 100,000.

Statistics from the Centers for Disease Control and Prevention (CDC) named suicide as the 11th-highest cause of death in 2005. Although the suicide rate has declined slightly among teens since 1992, it was the third-leading cause of death among young people ages 15 to 24 in 2005.

Completed suicides are only part of the problem. More people are hospitalized or treated and released as a result of suicide attempts than are fatally injured. While suicide is often viewed as a response to a single stressful event, it is a far more complicated issue.

CAUSES OF SUICIDE

Suicides are not caused by a single factor but by a combination of factors. **Depression** plays an important role in many suicides. About 75 percent of those who commit suicide are depressed. People often mistake depression for "feeling blue." Depression is more than a little sadness. It is caused by a number of factors ranging from chemical imbalances to environmental influences. A person with depression is likely to display one or more of the following behaviors:

- Feelings of worthlessness, hopelessness, helplessness, total indifference, or unreasonable guilt
- Prolonged sadness; unexplained crying spells
- Jumpiness or irritability
- Withdrawal from formerly enjoyable activities or relationships

- Inability to concentrate or remember details; indecisiveness
- Noticeable change in appetite with sudden weight loss or gain
- Changes in sleep patterns: constant fatigue, insomnia, early waking, oversleeping
- Physical ailments that cannot be otherwise explained

According to the Harris County Psychiatric Center at the University of Texas, other contributing factors to suicides and attempted suicides may include:

- Substance abuse
- Divorce of parents
- Parental unemployment
- Financial problems
- Isolation from family or friends
- Rejection by a boyfriend or girlfriend
- Domestic violence or abuse
- Lack of success at school

Q & A

Question: Aren't most suicides committed by women?

Answer: According to a 2009 fact sheet by the Centers for Disease Control, males represent 79 percent of all completed suicides. However, women are two to three times more likely than men to attempt suicide. Although more women try to commit suicide, significantly more men succeed at it.

PREVALENCE AMONG YOUNG PEOPLE

According to statistics published by the Centers for Disease Control and Prevention (CDC) on the major causes of death among young people, only unintentional injuries—mostly car crashes—and murder are responsible for more deaths among teens. Every two years since 1991, the CDC has conducted a nationwide survey of students in grades nine through 12 to assess attitudes that might affect their health. The Youth Risk Behavior Surveillance System (YRBSS) is a nationwide survey conducted every other year of students in grades nine through 12. In the 2007 YRBSS, 28.5 percent of the teens surveyed reported feeling sad or hopeless almost every day for two weeks. In the 12 months before the survey, 14.5 percent considered suicide. In that same time period, 11.3 percent of the students actually planned a suicide. Approximately half that number—6.9 percent—went as far as attempting to kill themselves.

Teens can be especially susceptible to suicidal thoughts. Adolescents experience dramatic biochemical changes. Sudden mood swings are common. As their sexuality emerges, teens are faced with new experiences, feelings, and challenges. These sometimes disorienting changes can be complicated by substance abuse.

The teen years are also often filled with intensive self-examination. Young people often ask themselves, "Who am I?" or "Why don't I fit in?" These questions can lead some people into despair, especially if they are already experiencing depression or other mental disorders.

Another element that makes being a teenager especially difficult is the realization that one is about to become an adult. As a child, one feels like an extension of his or her parents. As an adolescent, once-respected adults are now authority figures who seem to want the teenager to stay a child forever. Many wish their parents would do more than just tell them what they can't do. These changes in the relationship between teens and their parents can lead to heated discussions and disagreements. Hurt feelings on both sides are common and can cause emotional distress.

Some young people are idealistic. They have high moral and ethical standards that they would like everyone to live up to. Life is not perfect. Bad things happen. No one is perfect. People make mistakes. Those who are particularly idealistic may be disturbed or disappointed by life's ups and downs.

Community loss—the tragedy of September 11, the loss of the Columbia shuttle, the war in Afghanistan can have devastating effects. If a person is already feeling things are hopeless, it's easy to see tragedies as evidence that nothing and no one is safe.

SUICIDE INTERVENTION

The best time to intervene in suicidal behavior is before a person actually makes a physical attempt. An article published by the Centers for Disease Control and Prevention describes a number of programs that aim at suicide prevention.

Many programs use the concept of a **gatekeeper**, a person trained to recognize individuals who are at risk and offer help. At school, a gatekeeper could be a teacher, counselor, or coach. Some programs also teach these and other staff members how to deal with suicides and other crises at their schools. Gatekeepers can also be recruited from the community, including clergy, police, staff members at recreation facilities, and doctors and nurses who provide health care for young people.

Some programs are aimed directly at students. These programs alert them to the warning signs of a potential suicide and how to get help for themselves or others. Other programs are designed to help students feel better about themselves and improve their social skills.

Identifying young people at risk for suicide may require screening programs. Such efforts use questionnaires or other means to identify possible suicidal attitudes. Screening can also be used to track changes in outlook and behavior, or even to evaluate the effectiveness of other suicide prevention projects.

Peer support programs can be organized both inside and outside schools, allowing students or young people to work together, helping one another and learning to help themselves. Such programs may help to break the isolation often experienced by young people at risk. These programs may also help them learn better social skills.

The program most often featured in the media is the telephone hotline or crisis center. Here, trained volunteers and paid professional staff offer counseling over the phone or face-to-face. Such programs often include referrals to mental health services.

Access restriction programs seek to keep those who wish to take their own life from potential weapons such as guns, drugs, or poisons. Other programs offer a plan of action after a suicide has occurred. These responses are usually aimed at friends and relatives of those who have committed suicide. In part, the effort is to avoid suicide clusters—attempts to copy the initial suicide. In addition, these programs may help young people cope with their feelings of loss at the death of a friend or peer.

Fact Or Fiction?

Suicide victims are all wound up in their private little worlds.

The Facts: Suicide may be an intensely personal decision, but that decision is affected by events in the larger world. Suicide clusters occur when two or more individuals try to copy the suicide of someone they know or have heard about through media coverage. A 2001 article in the *British Journal of Psychology* discussed the reaction to the 1997 death of Princess Diana, a well-known public figure. Researchers examined suicide figures for the month following her funeral and compared them with suicide rates for the same period of time over the prior five years. They found 17.4 percent more suicides after the funeral, especially among women, with a total increase of 33.7 percent. Young women, ages 24 to 44, were especially affected, with a higher suicide rate of 45.1 percent.

RECOGNIZING THE SIGNS

Suicides do not happen without warning. Most people give clues or talk about their feelings before acting upon them. Recognizing and responding to these clues can prevent suicide attempts and death. Teens who are considering suicide are likely to:

- Talk about or seem preoccupied with death; say things like "My family would be better off without me" or "I wish I were dead"
- Lose interest in important or pleasurable activities
- Do poorly in school
- Show signs and symptoms of depression
- Give away important possessions, clean their rooms, and throw things away
- Neglect hygiene and self-care
- Withdraw from relationships, family, or friends
- Behave recklessly, take high risks
- Abuse drugs and/or alcohol

Everyone experiences difficulties in life and may show one or more of these behaviors. However, when these behaviors form a pattern, they should not be ignored. Often, having the opportunity to speak to a sympathetic listener can help prevent a suicide. Essentially, that is the principle behind suicide telephone hotlines.

If a friend or acquaintance speaks seriously about suicide, do not keep silent. Remain calm and recognize your friend's conversation for what it is—a plea for help. Do not attempt to solve the problem on your own. Express your concerns for your friend's safety or state of mind to a teacher or counselor.

For many, suicide is a particularly distressing form of violence. The waste of a life—especially a young life—by one's own hand has a tragic effect on those the suicide victim leaves behind. Educating oneself about suicide, participating in suicide intervention programs, and staying open to friends and peers can make a difference.

See also: Alcohol and Violence; Assault and Bullying; Media and Violence; School Violence; Teens and Violence

FURTHER READING

Crook, Marion. *Out of the Darkness: Teens Talk About Suicide.* Vancouver, Canada: Arsenal Pulp Press, 2004.
Nelson, Gary E. *A Relentless Hope: Surviving the Storm of Teen Depression.* Eugene, Oreg.: Cascade Books, 2007.
Wallerstein, Claire. *Teen Suicide.* Chicago: Heinemann Library, 2003.

■ TEENS AND VIOLENCE

The connection between teens and violence—crime, gang violence, or fights—has worried Americans for many years, as shown by extensive media coverage on the subject. A sharp increase approximately 20 years ago resulted in greater public awareness and concern. A 2001 special report by the surgeon general, the nation's highest-ranking public health officer, stated, "The epidemic of youth violence that began in 1983 and peaked in 1993 is not over. Arrest rates for violent crimes by youth have dropped significantly since 1993, giving cause for hope, but other indicators of violent behavior remain high."

The report cited three major reasons for the surge in violence: a growth in gang membership, involvement of young people in the sale of illegal drugs, and the use of guns.

The Centers for Disease Control and Prevention (CDC) described the impact of those factors in its 2001–2002 Injury Fact Book. It noted that teens and young adults tend to act impulsively and engage in risk-taking behaviors. Add a deadly weapon like a gun to impulsive behavior and the results can be extremely risky—even fatal.

VICTIMS OF VIOLENCE

According to the CDC, more than 720,000 young people ages 10 to 24 were injured from violent acts in 2006. One of the tools the government uses to assess dangers to young people is a national survey made every other year of students in grades nine to 12. Results of the 2007 Youth Risk Behavior Surveillance System (YRBSS) showed that 5.9 percent of the students surveyed had carried a weapon in the previous month, including 5.2 percent who had carried a gun, almost 36 percent of the students had gotten into a fight, and 4.2 of them were injured sufficiently enough that they needed medical treatment.

For several years, the CDC has identified homicide as the second-leading cause of death for people aged 15 to 24, and the leading cause of death for African Americans in the same age group. The Bureau of Justice Statistics reports that 16- to 19-year-olds are more likely than other Americans to experience a violent crime.

Examination of statistics for violent crimes in the National Crime Victimization Survey shows a similar pattern. People under the age of 24 are more likely to be victims of murder, rape, robbery, and aggravated assault than those who are over 24.

According to the Bureau of Justice Statistics, in 2006 teens experienced the highest rate of violent crime. In 2007, there was one rape or sexual assault for every 1,000 people ages 12 and higher. This number goes up to 3.4 per 1,000 for those ages 12 through 15, and 2.5 per 1,000 for teens between ages 16 and 19. There were also 39.6 assaults and 4.0 robberies per 1,000 adolescents ages 12 through 15. These figures rise to 44.7 and 4.6, respectively, for teens ages 16 through 19.

Dating violence victims

Dating violence refers to physical or sexual abuse by a date or acquaintance. It also includes verbal threats, intimidation, and emotional abuse. A 2001 article in the *Journal of the American Medical Association* stated that approximately 20 percent of adolescent girls have reported being physically or sexually hurt by a dating partner.

The 2007 Youth Risk Behavior Surveillance study indicates that 9.9 percent of students have been slapped, hit, or physically hurt by a dating partner. The report also indicates that 7.8 percent of students were forced to have sexual intercourse against their will.

Victims of bullying

The Center for the Study and Prevention of Violence at the University of Colorado at Boulder has identified two primary types of victims of bullying. First is the passive or submissive victim, and the second is called the provocative victim. Passive victims send out the message that they are weak or insecure and that they will probably not fight back if they are bullied. The provocative victim can be either anxious or aggressive in dealing with their classmates.

Fact Or Fiction?

Bullying is just a part of growing up.

The Facts: A study by the advocacy group Kids First found that children who had been bullied grow up to be sadder than others, with lower self-esteem. They have been known to turn violence inward by committing suicide and outward by harming others. Three-quarters of the young shooters in recent cases of school gun violence were victims of bullying.

Bullies face difficulties as adults as well. Scandinavian researchers, who were among the first to pay scientific attention to bullying, conducted a long-term study. By their mid-20s, young men who had been identified by classmates as bullies had significantly more trouble with the law. Among the former bullies, 60 percent had been convicted of a crime, compared to a crime rate of 23 percent among those who had not shown bullying behavior. In addition, 35 to 40 percent of the former bullies had three convictions, compared to only 10 percent of those in the non-bullying group.

The center lists the following characteristics for passive/submissive victims:

- Are physically weaker than their peers (particularly boys)
- Display "body anxiety." They are afraid of being hurt, have poor physical coordination, and are ineffective in physical play or sports
- Have poor social skills and have difficulty making friends
- Are cautious, sensitive, quiet, withdrawn, and shy
- Cry or become upset easily
- Are anxious, insecure, and have poor self-esteem
- Have difficulty standing up for or defending themselves in peer groups
- Relate better to adults than to peers

Provocative victims display these characteristics:

- Exhibit some or all of the characteristics of passive or submissive victims
- Are hot-tempered and attempt to fight back when victimized—usually not effectively
- Are hyperactive, restless, have difficulty concentrating, and create tension
- Are clumsy, immature, and exhibit irritating habits
- Are also disliked by adults, including teachers
- Try to bully students weaker than themselves

The experience of being bullied can have severe consequences. Victims may develop feelings of low self-worth and even turn to suicide.

Victims of hate crimes

Hate crimes are crimes prompted by an individual's race, religion, sexual orientation, gender, ethnic or national origin, or disability. These crimes aim to terrorize an entire community. In 2006, the Federal Bureau of Investigation's Uniform Crime Reporting program reported on 7,722 hate crimes. Approximately 60 percent of these were directed against an individual, including simple assault (without a weapon), aggravated assault, rape, and murder. Crimes against property (robbery, vandalism, destroying, stealing, or setting fire to vehicles, homes, stores, and places of worship) accounted for approximately 32 percent of these crimes. Additional forms of abuse included threats by mail, telephone, or e-mail.

Q & A

Question: Why do so many teens get involved with drugs and guns?

Answer: As the American Prosecutors Resource Institute points out, the involvement of young people in the drug trade resulted from a cold-blooded business decision by drug dealers. During the 1980s, many states adopted new laws with stern punishments for drug sales. Dealers began to recruit young people, who face less serious penalties in juvenile court. With the explosion in sales of crack, a cheap form of cocaine, many of these young "apprentices" started dealing themselves—and carrying guns to protect their merchandise and money.

PERPETRATORS OF VIOLENCE

According to the surgeon general's *Special Report on Youth Violence,* arrest rates for violent crimes have declined since 1994, primarily due to fewer young people using guns. A number of factors were cited as contributing to this reduction—a decline in youth involvement in the crack cocaine market, police crackdowns on gun carrying, a strong economy, and crime and violence prevention programs. However, many other indicators of youth violence remain high. Arrest rates for aggravated assaults are nearly 70 percent higher than they were in 1983, and self-reporting studies indicate that the proportion of young people involved in violent behavior and the rates of violent offending have not declined since the mid-1990s.

The National Center for Injury Prevention and Control has identified factors that put young people at risk for becoming violent. In general, adolescent males are much more likely to be violent than females. An early history of acting aggressively can predict later violence, especially if youthful violence involves **antisocial behavior**—a repeated pattern of disregard for and violation of the rights of others. Antisocial behavior often includes fighting, habitual lying, reckless disregard for the safety of others, and acts like setting fires or hurting animals. Another sign of later aggressiveness is the individual's belief that violence is acceptable behavior.

DID YOU KNOW?

Percentage of High School Students Who Carried a Gun or Other Weapon, by Ethnicity, Sex, and Grade

	Carried a Weapon			Carried a Gun		
	Female	Male	Total	Female	Male	Total
Race/Ethnicity						
White	6.5	29.3	18.6	1.5	9.5	5.8
Black	7.8	21.0	14.4	1.8	13.2	7.6
Hispanic	7.9	26.5	17.2	1.9	8.2	5.1
Grade						
9	7.6	27.3	18.0	1.4	9.8	5.9
10	7.2	28.5	18.4	1.8	9.9	6.1
11	6.3	25.6	16.2	1.7	8.9	5.4
12	6.4	26.5	16.6	1.6	10.6	6.2
Total	7.1	27.1	17.5	1.7	9.8	5.9

Source: Centers for Disease Control and Prevention, 2010.

Perpetrators of sexual violence in dating tend to believe that men are supposed to be independent and competitive and women dependent and supportive. Based on these beliefs, some young males may attempt to "prove their manhood" through violence and sexual conquests. They are likely to choose friends who are also sexually aggressive and accept the use of violence to resolve some relationship conflicts.

TEENS SPEAK

Just Business

Raul is 14 years old. He is presently in custody awaiting trial on drug possession charges.

"It started when I was 10 years old. This guy called Hitter used to come and watch us playing hoops. He'd pass me 50 bucks to hang and play ball. Everybody knew he was dealing—as his stuff looked fine.

"Soon I was helping him out—watching on the street for cops. Three hundred dollars a week, just for looking out for cops in their big old unmarked Chevies." He grins and shakes his head.

"After a while, I began selling on the street for Hitter. It was cool. Nobody paid much attention to me out there 'cause I'm kinda short and looked young. They all called me 'Baby Face.'"

"I was doing really well—six hundred a week in my pocket. Hitter started me moving some serious weight. I'd be carrying thirty grand worth of merchandise. That's when I got a gun."

Raul's round face goes tight and grim. "But now that the cops caught me with dope and a gun, they're talking about charging me as an adult. Even if I get lucky and they treat me like a kid, they're gonna ship me off someplace far away from the hood."

Suddenly, he looks very young. "And this is all I know."

Using alcohol and other drugs is highly related to violence, especially suicide. A study reported by the National Clearinghouse on Alcohol and Drug Information on shared characteristics of suicide victims found that 70 percent of these people abused alcohol or drugs. Having a history of bullying or being bullied is related to being violent. Many bullying victims consider suicide.

Youths who are poorly supervised at home or are exposed to violence are more likely to become violent themselves. Students who have lost interest in school or have experienced failure in school are also more likely to show violent behavior. Finally, adolescents who have access to firearms are more likely to use them to perpetrate violence.

The surgeon general's report on youth violence revealed several factors that can predict whether an adolescent will become violent. For teens between the ages of 12 and 14, weak connections to family and the community were strong predictors of violent behavior. Other strong predictors included having friends who had trouble in school or with the law and gang membership.

The National School Safety Center has offered a checklist of characteristics of students most likely to become violent at school. Their list is a result of tracking school-based violent incidents for more than 20 years. Characteristics include:

- History of tantrums and uncontrollable angry outbursts
- Resorting to name-calling, cursing, or abusive language
- Habitually making violent threats when angry
- Having previously brought a weapon to school
- Background of discipline problems at school
- Background of substance abuse or dependency
- Few or no close friends in peer group
- Preoccupation with weapons or explosives
- Displaying cruelty to animals
- Little or no adult supervision outside of school
- Witnessing or being a victim of neglect or abuse
- Having been bullied or bullying others
- Blaming others for problems in his/her life
- Preferring TV, movies, and games that have violent themes
- Preferring reading materials with violent themes
- Reflecting anger, frustration, and the dark side of life in school essays or writings
- Involvement in a gang or social group outside the peer norm
- Often feeling depressed or showing mood swings
- Threatening or attempting suicide

The teenage years are only a fraction of an American's potential lifespan of 70 years or more. Unfortunately, for too many young people this brief experience is colored by conflict. All they know is violence. The problem with following a violent lifestyle, however, is that it may be all too short, ending painfully and abruptly.

See also: Alcohol and Violence; Assault and Bullying; Media and Violence; School Violence

FURTHER READING

Barbour, Scott. *Teen Violence*. San Diego, Calif.: Greenhaven Press, 1999.

Fleeman, William. *Managing Teen Anger and Violence. A Pathway to Peace Program*. Manassas Park, Va.: Impact Publications, 2008.

■ TERRORISM

Planned acts of violence intended to kill, injure, and cause fear in as many people as possible. Terrorism is a worldwide problem today, with at least 11,800 terrorist attacks occurring in 2008. Cyberterrorism is one of the newer forms of terrorism, a result of the world's growing dependence on computers and the Internet. Currently, the United States is ill-prepared to handle cyberterrorist acts. Bioterrorism, another type of terrorism that has existed for centuries, is also a serious current threat, and one for which no nation is fully prepared to combat. Terrorist attacks, or the fear of such attacks, can lead to several emotional disorders, such as depression and anxiety.

WHAT IS TERRORISM?

Terrorism is easy to recognize and hard to define. If you examine the academic or research literature, there are numerous definitions. Government agencies around the world define terrorism differently. Terrorism involves the systematic threat or use of violence. This planned threat or use of violence is designed to kill, injure, or create fear in as many people as possible. The U.S. Federal Bureau of Investigation (FBI) defines terrorism as "the unlawful use of force or violence against persons or property to intimidate or coerce a government, the civilian population, or any segment thereof, in furtherance of political or social objectives."

In a 2009 report, the U.S. National Counterterrorism Center reported that there were approximately 11,800 terrorist attacks during 2008. The attacks took place around the world, with most occurring in the Middle East. The attacks resulted in more than 54,000 deaths, kidnappings, and injuries. Even though this is a horrifying number, it represents a decrease from the prior year. There was an 18 percent drop in the number of attacks from 2007, as well as 30 percent fewer deaths. During 2008, only 33 American deaths were reported, with the majority (21) occurring in Iraq.

Several types of terrorism exist. Conventional terrorism involves the use of bombs, kidnappings, attacks, suicide bombings, and hostage-taking, among other tactics. According to the World Health

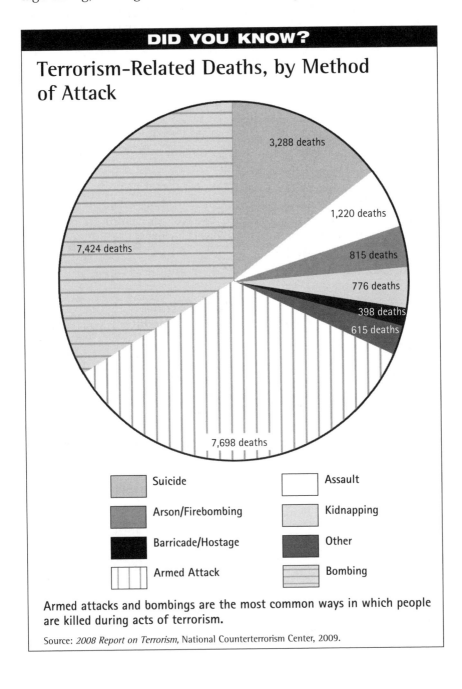

DID YOU KNOW?

Terrorism-Related Deaths, by Method of Attack

3,288 deaths

1,220 deaths

815 deaths

776 deaths

398 deaths

615 deaths

7,424 deaths

7,698 deaths

- Suicide
- Assault
- Arson/Firebombing
- Kidnapping
- Barricade/Hostage
- Other
- Armed Attack
- Bombing

Armed attacks and bombings are the most common ways in which people are killed during acts of terrorism.

Source: *2008 Report on Terrorism,* National Counterterrorism Center, 2009.

Organization (WHO), nuclear terrorism involves the use of nuclear weapons or highly radioactive sources. There have been no nuclear terrorist acts to date. However, this type of terrorism causes great concern because of the death and destruction nuclear weapons and radioactive materials can cause. Cyberterrorism and bioterrorism are two other types of terrorism. Because these types of attacks do not receive as much attention in the media as, for example, ecoterrorism (usually the destruction of property to support environmental causes), they are discussed in more detail here.

CYBERTERRORISM

Cyberterrorism, one of the newer forms of terrorism, is also known as information warfare. As the world relies more and more upon computers and the Internet, more opportunities arise for terrorists to cause damage and disrupt peoples' lives.

There are several definitions of cyberterrorism—from various organizations, experts, and government agencies. However, one definition stands out for its thoroughness. In May 2000, a computer scientist named Dorothy Denning provided a definition during her testimony before the House Armed Services Committee. According to that definition:

> Cyberterrorism is the convergence of cyberspace and terrorism. It refers to unlawful attacks and threats of attacks against computers, networks, and the information stored therein when done to intimidate or coerce a government or its people in furtherance of political or social objectives. Further, to qualify as cyberterrorism, an attack should result in violence against persons or property, or at least cause enough harm to generate fear. Attacks that lead to death or bodily injury, explosions, or severe economic loss would be examples. Serious attacks against critical infrastructures could be acts of cyberterrorism, depending on their impact. Attacks that disrupt nonessential services or that are mainly a costly nuisance would not.

PREVENTION OF CYBERTERRORISM

The Government Accountability Office (GAO) studied the government's ability to prevent cyber attacks. The GAO is an independent agency that works for Congress. The agency produces nonpartisan (neutral) research reports that have been requested by Congress. The agency evaluates the effectiveness of government programs, conducts policy analyses, examines how tax dollars are spent, and so forth. The

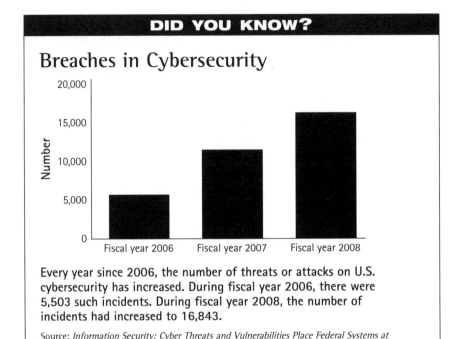

DID YOU KNOW?

Breaches in Cybersecurity

Every year since 2006, the number of threats or attacks on U.S. cybersecurity has increased. During fiscal year 2006, there were 5,503 such incidents. During fiscal year 2008, the number of incidents had increased to 16,843.

Source: *Information Security: Cyber Threats and Vulnerabilities Place Federal Systems at Risk,* Testimony Before the House Subcommittee on Government Management, Organization, and Procurement, Government Accountability Office, 2009.

work performed by the GAO is meant to be unbiased and informative and not to further any political agenda.

The GAO found that the federal government is not adequately prepared to stop cyber threats. The agency found widespread securities problems in the federal computer networks. As a result, financial and taxpayer information, security operations and procedures, medical records, and other data the federal government collects and maintains is at risk of being exposed.

There are several types of cyber attacks that can take place. One example is "denial of service." This type of attack can overwhelm a network or block traffic to it. As a result, people who have legitimate reasons to access information or services cannot do so. If you ever tried to make a call and received an automated, "All lines are busy. Please try later," message, or tried accessing a Web site only to receive a message that the server is busy, then you have experienced a denial of service. This does not mean that you experienced the effects of a cyber attack. Being denied service can occur for legitimate reasons, such as too many people trying to do the same task at the same time. However, the effect is the same: You are "locked out" until fewer people are using the service or the problem has been fixed.

Another type of attack is the "sniffer." This type of attack is more indirect. It occurs when a program is created to intercept data being exchanged online to look for specific information. For example, an attacker could be looking for passwords, bank account numbers, social security numbers, and other sensitive information. This attack can easily go unnoticed unless proper security protocols are in place. What makes this especially dangerous is that, by the time the sniffer is found and disabled, information may have already been passed to the attacker.

In an effort to help combat cyberterrorism and address security concerns, the Comprehensive National Cybersecurity Initiative (CNCI) was adopted in January 2008. The goal of the initiative is to better understand, anticipate, and develop defenses against cybersecurity threats. As a result of the initiative, the National Cyber Security Center (NCSC) was created within the Department of Homeland Security (DHS). According to the DHS, the NCSC coordinates and integrates information to help secure U.S. cyber networks and systems. The center is also charged with helping to develop and foster more collaboration among federal agencies.

Since the terrorist attacks of September 11, 2001, many national governments, including that of the United States, have been increasingly wary of cyberterrorism. If terrorist organizations were to acquire the skills necessary to gain control of utility networks that govern power grids, gas lines, or other parts of the national infrastructure, they could potentially cause widespread harm.

BIOTERRORISM

According to the Centers for Disease Control and Prevention (CDC), bioterrorist attacks involve "the deliberate release of viruses, bacteria, or other germs (agents) used to cause illness or death in people, animals, or plants." Agents can be natural or developed elements.

One of the most memorable examples of a bioterrorist act occurring in the United States comes from a series of anthrax attacks in 2001. On September 18, 2001, people started receiving letters that contained anthrax spores. Anthrax is an infection that is caused by the bacterium *Bacillus anthracis*. It is rare to see people infected with anthrax. The infection is not contagious, as to become infected people need to be directly exposed to the bacterial **spores.** Anthrax can be treated with antibiotics. There are three forms of anthrax infection: skin (cutaneous), gastrointestinal, and inhalation. A person can get a skin infection by touching animals with an anthrax infection or coming into contact with anthrax spores. A gastrointestinal infection typically occurs when someone eats undercooked meat containing anthrax spores. Finally, an inhalation infection occurs when someone breathes in anthrax spores.

According to the FBI, the 2001 attacks resulted in five deaths, with 17 more being infected but surviving an anthrax infection. Letters with anthrax spores had been sent to various media stations and two U.S. senators. It was not until 2008 that the FBI was able to press charges against a suspect for the attacks. However, the suspect committed suicide before he could be arrested.

LIVING WITH TERRORISM

The threat of terrorism is a fact of life. In the United States, terrorist acts are often unsuccessful. However, the fear of an attack is always present for many. Living with the fear of an attack, or the aftermath of an attack, can take a psychological toll on people.

Authors of a 2008 article that appeared in the *Journal of the American Academy of Child & Adolescent Psychiatry* examined how teenagers' social support systems helped protect against depression resulting from terrorism. The authors gathered data from seventh and eighth grade students in Israel. The study was conducted over a five-month period in a community repeatedly subjected to rocket attacks. The authors discovered that adolescents with stronger social support networks had lower levels of depression as a result of the repeated attacks.

COPING WITH 9/11

There has been a great deal of research on how people have coped with the attacks of September 11, 2001. A 2008 article in *Psychiatry* focused on the psychiatric consequences of the attacks on people who lived in New York City. The authors studied people who went to a medical clinic in northern Manhattan. Approximately 25 percent of the patients surveyed had indicated they knew someone who was killed in the terrorist attacks. A year after the attacks, almost 50 percent of patients who lost someone from the attacks met the criteria for a mental disorder. By comparison, almost 33 percent of patients who did not lose someone during the attacks met the criteria for a mental disorder. Major depression, anxiety, and post-traumatic stress were the most common disorders found.

A 2005 study in the *Archives of General Psychiatry* focused on the effects of 9/11 on schoolchildren in grades four through 12. The data collected was not extensive enough to determine whether children suffered any psychiatric disorders resulting from the terrorist attacks. Instead, the authors were able to determine whether any "probable" disorders existed (whether evidence existed that a disorder may be present). It was found that agoraphobia (fear of being outside one's home), separation anxiety, and post-traumatic stress disorder were the most common probable disorders among schoolchildren. Overall, 28.6 percent of schoolchildren showed signs of at least one probable mental disorder. An interesting finding was that a child's direct exposure to the attacks was less important than the family's exposure to the attacks. In other words, having family members who were traumatized by the attacks played a stronger role than having been directly exposed to the attacks. Although the authors were unsure why this was the case, it proved to be one more important piece of information that helped counselors to determine if children were suffering from a mental disorder.

See also: Hate Crimes; Revenge, Cycle of; Violence Against Populations; War; Weapons of Violence.

FURTHER READING:

Chaliand, Gérard, and Arnaud Blin, eds. *The History of Terrorism: From Antiquity to al Qaeda.* Berkeley, Calif.: University of California Press. 2007.

Hoffman, Bruce. *Inside Terrorism.* New York: Columbia University Press, 2006.

Post, Jerrold M. *The Mind of the Terrorist: The Psychology of Terrorism from the IRA to al-Qaeda.* New York: Palgrave Macmillan, 2008.

■ VICTIMIZATION

See: Social Costs of Violence

■ VIOLENCE, CYCLE OF
See: Family Violence; Revenge, Cycle of

■ VIOLENCE, RANDOM
See: Communities and Violence

■ VIOLENCE AGAINST POPULATIONS

Prejudice-driven violence occurs against members of a group targeted specifically because they belong to that group. Racial, ethnic, and religious groups have historically been targets of violence. The motivation to attack such groups is based on prejudice. Those who commit these violent attacks see certain groups, such as sexual minorities, as threats and become motivated to reduce or eliminate the threats.

Hate crimes are the most common forms of violence against specific populations. Genocide is an extreme form of violence designed to completely eliminate a group and any of its supporters.

MOTIVATIONS TO COMMIT VIOLENCE

There are many reasons, in general, to commit violence. However, when violence is targeted against a specific population, prejudice plays a central role. In a 2008 article in the *Journal of Social Issues,* the author examined the role prejudice plays in violence against members of other groups, and, not surprisingly, discovered that a person's prejudice strongly influences the probability of using violence against others. Two factors were found to influence prejudice. The first is a person's belief that the other group poses a threat. The threat could be real or perceived. The threat can be economic, religious, political, and so forth.

Second, the amount of contact a person has with members of other groups negatively influences prejudice. In other words, the more contact a person has with members of a group, the lower his or her prejudice will be. Being around members of other groups helps break down any **stereotypes** that may be perceived. When we know members of groups frequently targeted, it is easier to view them as people, rather than as outsiders or threats or "those people."

In an article that appeared in a 2007 issue of *Identity: An International Journal of Theory and Research,* the author looked at how people can allow violence to occur against other groups. The author's focus was on genocide; however, some of his conclusions apply to discrimination and prejudice in general.

One way that people commit violence against others without feeling guilty is to dehumanize the targeted group. This means that members

---

DID YOU KNOW?

Violence and Hate Crimes

Percent of victimizations by types of crime

Type of Crime	Hate	Other than hate
Total	100.0%	100.0%
Violent Crime	83.7	22.9
Rape/sexual assault	4.0	1.0
Robbery	5.0	2.5
Aggravated assault	18.5	4.5
With injury	5.0	1.4
Threatened with weapon	13.5	3.1
Simple assault	56.2	15.0
With injury	10.6	3.5
Without injury	17.6	5.5
Verbal threat	28.0	6.0
Personal larceny	0.0%	0.7%
Household crime	16.3%	76.4%
Burglary	3.7	13.3
Motor vehicle theft	0.3	4.1
Theft	12.3	59.0

Hate crimes are much more likely to be violent crimes than non–hate crimes. As this chart shows, crimes not motivated by hate are primarily property crimes. Hate crimes, on the other hand, are personal.

Source: Hate Crimes Reported by Victims and Police. Bureau of Justice Statistics, 2005.

of the targeted group are considered to be subhuman or nonhuman. As a result, there are no moral obstacles to harming members of this group. Without the usual restrictions, there is no reason to refrain from hurting others. According to the author, one way to dehumanize others is by using language that reflects subhuman status, such as "maggots," "vermin," or "parasites."

"Moral justification" is another way to legitimize violence against a population. In an important 2002 article in the *Journal of Moral Education,* the author discussed the various ways that people "disengage" their morals, which allows them to overcome objections about harming others. Moral justification is seen as "acting for the greater good." Violence against others, specifically groups that are seen as threats, is considered acceptable because the violence is thought to reduce the threat.

VIOLENCE AGAINST LGBT POPULATIONS

One population often subjected to violence is the lesbian-gay-bisexual-transgendered (LGBT) population. The latest hate crimes data provided by the Bureau of Justice Statistics indicate that 18 percent of hate crimes are motivated because of a person's sexual orientation. Slightly more than 16 percent of male hate-crimes victims indicated that they were attacked because of their sexual orientation. Almost 20 percent of female hate crimes victims indicated that their sexual orientation was the reason for their being attacked.

In a 2009 article in *Aggression and Violent Behavior,* the author examined violence against transgendered people. According to the author, sexual assault and rape are the most documented forms of violence against those who are transgendered. In fact, approximately 50 percent of transgendered people have been the victims of unwanted sex. Some evidence indicates the majority of attacks were motivated by either homophobia or transphobia.

A 2007 report by the Virginia Department of Public Health examined various health and life-course experiences of transgendered residents of Virginia, including data on violence against those who are transgendered. Forty percent of those participating in the study said they had been physically attacked. Almost one-third (30 percent) revealed that they had been attacked between three and five times. The most common offender was a stranger, with 47 percent of the victims indicating that they had not known the attacker. The report also indicates that 27 percent of transgendered Virginians were the victims of sexual assault, with strangers committing the assault in 27 percent of the cases.

Similar findings were reported in a 2008 study in the *Journal of Interpersonal Violence*. In this study, the author examined the experiences of those who are gay, lesbian, or bisexual. Compared to the prior study in Virginia, only 13.1 percent of the people in this study were the targets of violence because of their sexual orientation. More than 12 percent of people reported having had objects thrown at them, while 23.4 percent had been threatened with violence. Gay men were the most likely to be targets of violence, with 24.9 percent being victims of violent behavior.

VIOLENCE AGAINST RACIAL GROUPS

U.S. history is rife with incidents of violence committed against racial groups, in particular against African Americans. One of the more infamous examples is the enactment of Jim Crow laws. These were laws designed to keep blacks subservient to whites. In the 19th century, slavery had been abolished, and Jim Crow legislation was intended to prevent newly freed slaves from truly being free or equal to whites. Some of the restrictions placed on blacks by these laws included not being allowed to eat with whites, not being allowed to shake hands with whites, not being allowed to show any sign of public affection, not being allowed to curse at whites, and being required to use titles for whites, although whites did not have to reciprocate.

Although the laws themselves were not violent, violence was used to enforce them. A common means of enforcing the laws and maintaining social control was to lynch blacks. Mobs would track down, viciously beat, and then hang blacks in public. Lynchings could occur for any reason—if a black person spoke in the wrong tone, looked at someone "inappropriately," or tried to vote. Lynchings were intended to send a terrifying message to blacks not to cause problems or challenge existing conventions. While it is not possible to know the exact numbers, it is estimated that more than 3,000 blacks were lynched between 1882 and 1968.

Although Jim Crow laws were dismantled, and the Civil Rights movement of the 1960s helped black Americans obtain equal rights, violence continued. Assassination was used in some parts of the country to try to intimidate blacks. One example is the murder of Medgar Evers, a black activist who fought for equal rights. He played a role in

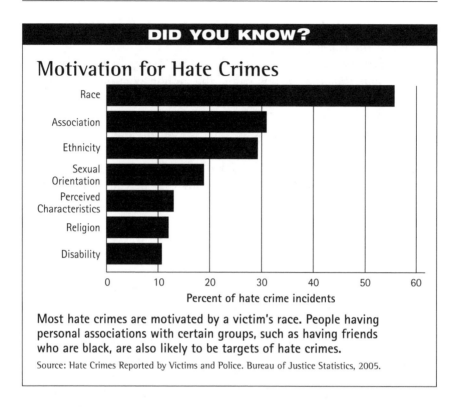

DID YOU KNOW?

Motivation for Hate Crimes

Percent of hate crime incidents

Most hate crimes are motivated by a victim's race. People having personal associations with certain groups, such as having friends who are black, are also likely to be targets of hate crimes.

Source: Hate Crimes Reported by Victims and Police. Bureau of Justice Statistics, 2005.

boycotting white businesses, as well as in helping to desegregate the University of Mississippi. Attempts were made on his life, and on June 12, 1963, he was shot in the back of the head. Less than an hour later, he died from the wound. It was not until 1994, 31 years later, that a member of the Klu Klux Klan, an organized white supremacist group, was found guilty of Evers's murder.

Probably the most infamous assassination was that of the Reverend Dr. Martin Luther King, Jr. Dr. King was considered one of the most prominent civil rights leaders of the black community. His work to end racial discrimination and segregation earned him a Noble Peace Prize in 1964. He did not believe in using violence to achieve equality. On April 4, 1968, Dr. King was in Memphis, Tennesee, to give a speech. He was on the second floor balcony of the hotel he was staying at when he was shot. Just over an hour later, he was officially declared dead from the wounds he received. His death sparked riots across the country.

Racial violence continues today. Crimes that are motivated by hate toward a group are now considered hate crimes, and according to the Bureau of Justice Statistics, blacks are the most common target of hate crimes motivated by race.

In a 2008 study in the journal *Social Forces,* the author examined the geography of hate crimes—against both blacks and whites. The idea was to see whether migration patterns into neighborhoods influenced racial violence. In other words, the author wanted to know if violence against blacks increased as blacks moved into predominately white neighborhoods. The author found that, indeed, hate crimes against blacks increased if blacks began to move into white neighborhoods where existing residents were similar to one another. As with other forms of violence against blacks, such as lynching and assassinations, these hate crimes were seen as a way to maintain the social order and keep blacks out of predominately white neighborhoods.

GENOCIDE

The most extreme form of violence against populations is genocide. According to the 1948 Convention on the Prevention and Punishment of Genocide, genocide is defined as any of the following acts committed with intent to destroy, in whole or in part, a national, ethnical, racial, or religious group: killing members of a group, inflicting serious mental or bodily harm, imposing measures intended to prevent birth within the group, transferring children of the group to other groups, and inflicting conditions of life, or deliberately depriving people of the resources they need to survive, on the group to destroy them.

The most infamous example of genocide is the Jewish Holocaust, in which the Nazis, led by the German dictator Adolf Hitler, systematically murdered Jews during the 1930s through the mid-1940s. More than 6 million Jews and an estimated 5 million more people were brutally killed during these years before and during World War II. Innocent victims were shot, burned, gassed, and exposed to a variety of lethal conditions while imprisoned in concentration and extermination camps with subhuman conditions.

Genocide is not a thing of the past. In 1994, there were an estimated 800,000 to 1.7 million people murdered during the "ethnic cleaning" that occurred in the African state of Rwanda. Two groups of citizens were targeted. The Tutsi citizens were the primary targets. They were viewed as enemies of the other main group of Rwandan citizens, the Hutu. The Tutsi were seen as oppressors who needed to be exterminated. Members of the Hutu who sympathized with the Tutsi were also targeted for murder. By wiping out one population and its sympathizers, members of the Hutu felt they could "reestablish" their rightful place in the country.

Another horrific example of ethnic cleansing took place in Bosnia during the early 1990s. The country formerly known as Yugoslavia was separated into several smaller countries. This created conflicts among the different groups of people who had lived in Yugoslavia: the Serbians, Croatians, and Albanians. Serbians are Orthodox Christians; Croatians are Catholics; and Albanians are Muslims. Acts of genocide were committed by the Serbs against the Albanians. Although an estimated 200,000 deaths occurred as a result of the civil conflict, other countries and the United Nations were hesitant to intervene. It was not until an incident occurred in which approximately 8,000 men and boys were murdered that the United States and NATO finally stepped in.

At the time of this writing (2009), another genocide is occurring, in the African nation of Sudan. A civil war in the Darfur region of Sudan began in 2003. Darfur ethnic groups—the Fur, Massalit, and Zhagawa—have been targeted by the Sudanese military and a militia called the Janjaweed. Approximately 300,000 Darfurians have been murdered, with more than 2.5 million being displaced from their homes. Women and girls have been primary targets of the military and militia. Raping and sexually assaulting women and girls is an effective way of destroying them and their families. Violence against entire populations—motivated by one type of prejudice or another—is a modern problem.

See also: Gang Violence; Hate Crimes; Terrorism; War

FURTHER READING

Ehrlich, Howard. *Hate Crimes and Ethnoviolence: The History, Current Affairs, and Future of Discrimination in America.* Boulder, Colo.: Westview Press.

Kiernan, Ben. *Blood and Soil: A World History of Genocide and Extermination from Sparta to Darfur.* New Haven, Conn.: Yale University Press. 2009.

■ VIOLENCE AND VIDEO GAMES

Relationship between video game violence—such as in Mortal Kombat—and violent behavior. For more than 25 years, there has been growing concern that the violent actions depicted in video games can lead to violent behavior by those who play the games. Most research indicates there is a link between playing violent video games and actual aggression or violence. However, most studies have examined this connection indirectly, with very few studies looking at playing violent video games and the actual behavior of people who play them.

PLAYING VIDEO GAMES

A brief report published in 2006 by the Federal Trade Commission cited data indicating that 83 percent of children between the ages of eight and 18 live in homes with a video game console. According to a 2008 report by the Entertainment Software Association, people in 65 percent of households in the United States play either video or computer games. Surprisingly, the association indicates that the average age of a video game player is 35.

A ratings system exists for video games. It was established by the Entertainment Software Rating Board (ESRB) and has two parts: a rating symbol and content descriptors. There are seven ratings symbols:

- AO—Adults Only;
- M—Mature;
- T—Teen;
- E10+—Everyone 10 and older;
- E—Everyone;
- EC—Early Childhood;
- RP—Rating Pending.

There are 32 different descriptors that can be used to indicate the content of the video game. Some of them include: Animated Blood, Blood, Blood and Gore, Intense Violence, and Sexual Themes. The goal of these ratings and descriptors is to help parents determine which games they are comfortable allowing their children to play.

VIOLENT VIDEO GAMES AND VIOLENT BEHAVIOR

There is some question as to whether playing violent video games influences actual violent behavior by game players. Most of the research indicates that playing these games does influence attitudes toward violence and the likelihood of engaging in violent behavior. For example, the authors of a 2007 study in the *Journal of Experimental Social Psychology* examined whether video game violence causes people to become desensitized to real-life violence. In this study, the authors discovered that playing violent video games for only 20 minutes can cause people to become less sensitized to real violence.

The process of desensitization is not unique to violence. Mental-health counselors often use behavioral therapies that help people become desensitized to anxiety-provoking stimuli. Exposure therapy is specifically designed to help eliminate emotional reactions. If desensitization occurs from playing violent video games, gamers can witness or engage in violence without any emotional reactions, such as shock, horror, or anxiety.

Violent video games may have more impact on people than watching violence in the media. People play video games, which requires involvement. Watching television, on the other hand, is more passive. One element of involvement deals with the realism of the games. The authors of a 2008 study in *Media Psychology* wanted to see if the quality of violent video games influenced subsequent actual anger and aggression. Over the years, the quality of games has increased: Graphics and sounds are much more realistic. With that being the case, it may be possible that more realistic video violence can have a greater impact on actual aggression and desensitization. While the authors found that video game quality did *not* have this impact, the amount of exposure does play an important role.

Q & A

Question: Can people become addicted to video games?

Answer: Although there is no definitive research, a survey was conducted in 2007 by the company HarrisInteractive, a market research firm, that indicated that video game addiction is a problem. The survey found that approximately 8.5 percent of video gamers from ages eight to 18 could be classified as having an addiction. Being addicted to video games means more than playing them all of the time. Addiction is evident when playing video games interferes with and damages a person's life. This survey found that those who can be classified as having an addiction to video games were more likely than others to have attention deficit problems, perform worse in school, and spend almost 25 hours playing games every week. That is the equivalent of working a part-time job, where someone makes a contribution and usually receives a salary.

The authors of a 2008 study in *Pediatrics* examined the effects video games have on children over time. In particular, the authors looked at aggressive behaviors of adolescents in the United States and Japan. It was found that constantly playing violent video games leads to a greater likelihood of being physically aggressive months later, compared to those who do not play violent games. This finding was consistent for adolescents in both the United States and Japan, despite significant cultural differences. The authors also discovered that the influence of violent video games on aggressive behavior was stronger in younger children. A possible explanation is that the longer children play violent video games, the greater the odds are of their engaging in aggressive behavior at some point.

Not everyone believes that video game violence influences real violence. Critics believe that aggressive individuals are naturally drawn to violent games. Any relationship that exists between video games and violent behavior is a result of some underlying character-istics of people who play those games and act aggressively toward other people.

An article published in a 2008 issue of *Criminal Justice and Behavior* examined the relationship between playing violent video games and actual violent behavior. The authors looked at play-ing habits and how often people engaged in violent or aggressive behavior. At first, a relationship was found between the two: Playing violent video games was related to violent and aggressive behavior. However, the authors found the relationship disappeared once other factors were taken into consideration. When the authors included "aggressive personality" and "exposure to family violence" in their statistics, the relationship between video game violence and actual violent behavior disappeared. In other words, the relationship can be considered a "by-product" of other factors, such as personality and family violence.

The authors of a 2007 study in the *Journal of Research in Personality* conducted a different type of study, to see whether a person's anger is more important than his or her exposure to violent video games. As with other studies, the authors found that people who played violent games showed increased signs of aggression compared to those who played nonviolent video games. It was also discovered that people with angrier personalities showed higher levels of aggression after playing violent games. The results of this study help verify that both personality characteristics and environmental influences (including exposure to media violence) play important roles in actual violent behavior.

In another study, in 2008, reported in the *Journal of Adolescent Research,* the authors interviewed 42 boys between the ages of 12 and 14 to obtain their opinions on video games. They found that the boys understood the difference between real violence and violence in video games. According to the authors, the boys played violent video games to express fantasies of glory and power. Another common theme was that the boys played games to alleviate stress and anger. There was no indication, however, that playing violent video games influenced their actual behavior.

VIOLENT VIDEO GAMES AND THE BRAIN

Although there is some question as to whether playing violent video games contributes to actual violent behavior, research has consistently shown that playing these games has at least a temporary effect on the brain. A 2006 article in the *Journal of Experimental Social Psychology* indicates that exposure to video game violence leads to being desensitized to real violence. The authors found that exposure to violent video games causes parts of the brain to slow down. These parts are important for emotions: It was discovered that there was very little emotional arousal when viewing the video games. In other words, those who played violent video games did not have as strong a reaction when viewing real violence. The authors discovered this because participants in the study were connected to an electrophysiological recording device, which allows researchers to monitor electrical activity in the brain.

The author of a 2005 article in the journal *Child Adolescent Psychiatric Clinics of North America* reviewed several effects that video game violence has on people, particularly adolescents. One area the author mentions is the impact that playing video games has on the brain. Exposure to violence, including media and video game violence, alters how the brain interprets events. The concept of desensitization is not only psychological. In a sense, the brain reorganizes itself and no longer processes this information as "shocking" or "disruptive."

Media violence, including video game violence, has been shown to affect how the brain functions. In a 2007 article in *Current Directions in Psychological Science,* the authors conducted a review of studies to see how media violence influences brain and body functioning. One

finding they comment on is the role that the brain plays in desensitization. When people are exposed to violent media, including video games, parts of the brain that inhibit aggressive behavior are not as active. That is, the brain no longer works as hard to prevent aggressive behavior from happening.

A 2006 study in *Human Brain Mapping* presented findings of brain imaging of people while playing violent video games. The authors of the study report that exposure to violent video games at least temporarily alters brain functioning. In particular, those parts of the brain that focus on empathy and on helping to regulate aggressive behavior become suppressed.

Q & A

Question: Can laws be passed to help regulate violent video games?

Answer: There have been attempts to regulate violent video games. In 2005, the California assembly passed the "ultra-violent video games bills," which were then signed into law by the governor. One bill called for banning the sales of these video games to minors. The other bill mandated that games rated "mature" be separated from other games. This bill also required stores to display the video game rating system established by the ESRB. However, in 2009, a U.S. court of appeals found these laws unconstitutional because video games are a form of free speech that cannot be censored without proper justification. In this case, the state did not provide enough justification that violent video games cause harm to children. Issues of regulation continue to be debated.

See also: Gang Violence; Media and Violence

FURTHER READING

Kutner, Lawrence, and Cheryl Olson. *Grand Theft Childhood: The Surprising Truth About Violent Video Games and What Parents Can Do.* New York: Simon & Schuster, 2008.

Loguidice, Bill, and Matt Barton. *Vintage Games: An Insider Look at the History of Grand Theft Auto, Super Mario, and the Most Influential Games of All Time.* St. Louis, Mo.: Focal Press, 2009.

■ VIOLENT BEHAVIOR, CAUSES OF

Factors that may influence a person to act aggressively. The causes of violence seem to relate to genetics, family influence, social skill development, psychological impairments, hormones, steroids, and social influences.

HEREDITARY INFLUENCES

To answer the question of whether violent behavior is inherited, scientists must establish the existence of a specific **gene** that makes some people violent and others nonviolent. Present estimates suggest that a human has between 28,000 and 120,000 genes. No one has found real evidence to date that a single gene or combination of genes predicts violent behavior.

Evidence does exist suggesting that one's genetic makeup does predict some aspects of one's personality. Humans may inherit personality traits that make them more prone to violent behavior under certain conditions. The idea, however, that a single gene causes someone to be violent is not supported by research.

Fact Or Fiction?

Youth violence isn't a problem. The crime rate is going down.

The Facts: Rates for violent crime, specifically homicide, have dropped. That decline is mainly in gun-related violence, which rose sharply in the mid-1990s. Analysis of FBI crime reports shows that once gun-related cases are removed, rates of violent crime are relatively unchanged over a 20-year period.

LEARNED OR ENVIRONMENTAL INFLUENCES

Because no direct link between genes and violence has been discovered, researchers think environment plays an important role in determining whether people become violent. In a sense, violence is a learned behavior.

In 1999, Laurence Steinberg, a social scientist who studies violent behavior, addressed the Working Group on Youth Violence established by the U.S. House of Representatives. Steinberg identified family relationships as the major factor in predicting mental health problems among children and adolescents. Parents who show hostility toward their children or who neglect them create young people at risk for mental problems. These problems may lead to antisocial behaviors, a disregard for the rights of others, persistent violations of rules, and ultimately to violence.

When young children experience or witness violence in their homes or neighborhoods, they learn to associate all conflict of any sort with violence. For them, violence becomes the first response to disagreement or frustration. They come to regard aggressiveness as accepted, even normal behavior. As they grow older, acting on aggressive impulses may lead to violent and even criminal behavior.

Steinberg was involved in a 10-year study of 20,000 adolescents. According to a 2000 issue of the *National Institute of Justice Journal,* he and other researchers found that students who experienced the most problems with school, friends, violence, or the law had parents who were not involved in their children's lives.

A 1997 article in the *Journal of Children and Society* reported similar findings, based on interviews with young offenders. The young offenders described seeing their parents display poor judgment and violent behavior in relationships. They also admitted feeling unloved, neglected, and not understood by their parents. As Dr. Steinberg explained in his congressional testimony, for parents to successfully rear children who become healthy adults, the children must be the priority.

PSYCHOLOGICAL IMPAIRMENTS

Certain patterns of behavior suggest that aggressive individuals face some psychological challenges. In a 1997 study in the journal *Suicide and Life Threatening Behavior,* researchers determined that adolescents hospitalized for aggression or attempted suicide were more likely to have unrealistic views of their health. Their anxiety and levels of fear were abnormally high. Many suffered from paranoia, a psychological disorder characterized by feelings of persecution, and early stages of schizophrenia, a psychological disorder characterized by a distorted sense of reality. They also suffered from social introversion, a tendency to shrink from social contacts. These diagnoses have become important in predicting whether a person will turn violence inward by harming themselves or turn it outward by striking out against others.

A 2009 study in the *Archives of General Psychiatry* focused on the link between mental disorders and violence. The authors found that those with mental disorders had slightly more violent incidents that those without such disorders. That finding alone was not enough to conclude with any confidence that individuals with mental disorders are more likely to engage in violent behaviors. However, the authors did find that those with mental disorders and substance abuse or dependence issues were significantly more likely to engage in violent behavior. Results of the study also indicated that 46 percent of those with a mental disorder also had a history of substance abuse or dependence.

A 1992 article in *Phi Delta Kappan* magazine identified a series of nonclinical psychological factors that may influence how aggressive an individual becomes. These included lower levels of intelligence, shyness, acting out as a response to frustration, and an inability to set goals.

Psychological problems can impact other factors to result in an act of violence whether or not a clinical diagnosis exists. The environment again plays a major role in the act of violence. For instance, many people have difficulty setting goals. Not all of them become violent. In fact, only a small percentage does. Those who act out their frustrations do so when they find themselves in unfamiliar or uncomfortable situations. At that point, their inability to set a goal is magnified by their frustration at not meeting some level of expectation, real or imagined. People who have developed social skills and skills in anger management can work through conflict, while for those whose skills are less developed, conflict may become violent.

DEFICIENT SOCIAL SKILLS

An individual's inability to manage conflict often serves as the trigger for an act of violence. No one can avoid conflict entirely. Everyone needs the skills necessary to negotiate tension without violence. Those skills are learned. They include the ability to become closely associated with others, to communicate, control one's anger, cooperate, ask for help when needed, and delay personal gratification.

A 1996 article in *Elementary School Guidance and Counseling* identified the importance of the following skills in addressing aggressive responses in youths:

- Problem solving: the ability to identify the conflict at hand, see a variety of solutions, and choose the one best suited for the situation

- Anger control: the ability to control internal (thought-oriented) anger and external (actions toward others) anger when the time arises through positive self-talk and such physical actions as deep breathing, counting, or walking away.

- Assertiveness: standing up for oneself in situations where one's rights may be violated, but doing so in such a way that one doesn't violate the rights of others

HORMONAL AND BIOLOGICAL INFLUENCES

The idea that there may be a chemical link to violent behavior has received growing support in the scientific community. The human body contains many chemicals, including **hormones,** substances that initiate and stop body processes and even emotions. A hormonal imbalance can affect a person's mood and emotions.

In her 1996 article on the causes of violence printed in *Elementary School Guidance and Counseling,* Jeannine Studer points out that the hormones **serotonin** and testosterone may affect violent behaviors. Serotonin is a chemical the brain uses to regulate mood. Low levels of serotonin are most often associated with depression. The relationship between violence and serotonin has been researched in both humans and nonhuman subjects. The possibility of violent behaviors seems to be elevated in individuals who have low levels of serotonin. The low levels impact their ability to manage emotions (like depression and anger).

Testosterone is a hormone connected with sex differences. The reason men tend to be more aggressive than women is often attributed to the higher levels of testosterone in men. Studer notes, however, that low levels of serotonin and high levels of testosterone in and of themselves do not predict violence. Environmental factors usually trigger violent acts, and abnormal levels of these two hormones may make some people more likely to physically express their anger.

Steroids are hormonelike substances chemically similar to testosterone. Androgenic steroids are actually based on testosterone, while anabolic steroids are synthetic forms of the hormone. Testosterone, of course, has been linked with the higher levels of aggressiveness in males. By dosing themselves with steroids in the hope of increasing muscle mass and endurance, men magnify the amount of testosterone in their system. Such magnification increases the degree of aggression in individuals taking the drug.

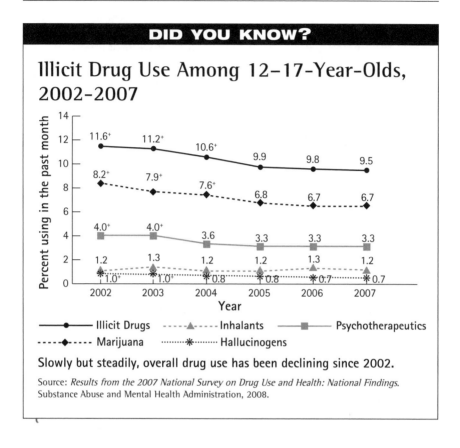

DID YOU KNOW?

Illicit Drug Use Among 12-17-Year-Olds, 2002-2007

Slowly but steadily, overall drug use has been declining since 2002.

Source: *Results from the 2007 National Survey on Drug Use and Health: National Findings.* Substance Abuse and Mental Health Administration, 2008.

The Monitoring the Future survey, a yearly poll conducted by the National Institute on Drug Abuse (NIDA), tracks the growth in steroid use. In 2007, the survey reported that 1.5 percent of eighth graders, 1.8 percent of 10th graders, and 2.2 percent of 12th graders had used steroids at some point in their lives. However, since steroid use is illegal, the real percentage may be much higher.

A survey by the Centers for Disease Control and Prevention (CDC) of high school students in Louisiana found that 12 percent of the boys and 5.7 percent of the girls used steroids. In establishing a campaign against steroid abuse, the head of the NIDA estimated that about 500,000 eighth and 10th graders used these performance-enhancing drugs. The University of Michigan Health System claims that at least 1 million Americans have tried steroids.

Steroids have serious side effects. In men, they can cause liver and kidney damage, development of breasts, acne, baldness, cysts, sterility, and reduced sex drive. In women, steroid use can prevent pregnancy, cause breasts to atrophy, develop menstrual irregularities, and develop male-pattern baldness and the deepening of the voice.

Another side effect of the drug is sudden outbursts of anger, or what is commonly referred to as **steroid rage.** Researchers have yet to figure out who is most likely to be affected by this side effect, or even what levels of steroid use will trigger rage.

A 1996 article published in the *Medical Journal of Australia* identified some of the changes that occur at varying levels of steroid use. In the early stages of use confidence, energy, and self-esteem all seemed to increase. Some athletes notice an ability to train despite pain, and even experience an increase in sex drive, but often report an overriding sense of irritation or edginess. As use continues over time and dosages increase, the Australian researchers noticed that users were less likely to show good judgment and were more likely to be impulsive. They also noted an increase in paranoid thoughts and aggressive behavior.

At high dosage levels, the Australian researchers found, users became very aggressive, hostile, violent, and uncontrolled—a danger to themselves and others. In other words, they displayed the signs of steroid rage. These outbursts of anger resulted in property damage, injuries to the users (including reckless driving or crashing cars), assaults, family and intimate violence, child abuse, suicide, and attempted murder or murder.

Another 1996 study refuted these conclusions. Researchers found no change in mood among the 43 men they followed in a clinically controlled study. Each man received 600 milligrams of testosterone each week for 10 weeks. According to the *New England Journal of Medicine,* the researchers measured changes in each subject's strength and whether he became more hostile or easily angered. While they found no change in mood, the researchers admitted that the amount of performance-enhancing drug given was controlled, and the men were screened in advance. If a steroid user was unstable to begin with or took large, uncontrolled dosages, rage was possible. The 600 milligrams of testosterone given the men in the study was six times the normal levels of testosterone in males. However, athletes who use steroids use 10 to 40 times their normal testosterone level, or 4,000 milligrams a week.

Because every individual's body chemistry is different, responses to performance-enhancing drugs may vary. However, the length of time people use steroids and the dosage they take seem to work together to cause the greatest negative effect and the most likely trigger for violent behavior.

Q & A

Question: Don't video games have a rating system to make sure violent games don't wind up in the hands of kids?

Answer: The National Institute on Media and the Family surveyed 778 students, grades four through 12 about video games in 2003. The average age of the young people was 13.5. Some 87 percent of the boys played M-rated games, which are supposedly restricted to players 17 and older. When asked to name their favorite games, 78 percent of the boys listed M-rated games in their top five, and 40 percent said that their favorite game was rated M.

These statistics suggest that many stores are not enforcing the ratings system. Nor are parents doing so. One out of five of the boys in the survey admitted to buying an M-rated game without parental permission.

SOCIETAL INFLUENCE

Social scientists continue to debate whether watching violence in the movies or on TV or reading about it causes a person to act violently. If there were a direct link between the two, wouldn't everyone who watched a violent action film leave the theater and engage in fights, if not murder? As with so many causes of violence, the answer seems to lie in a combination of individual factors, including an individual's predisposition to violence, whether he or she has a nonmedicated mental illness, and the immediate environment.

Many fear that viewing many acts of violence can have a desensitizing effect on individuals, especially young people. Given the amount of violence on the air, some estimate that by the time teens finish high school, they will have seen over 100,000 acts of violence on network television. If they have access to cable television, as most do today, that number is probably much higher.

Video games have also become a regular means of entertainment for youths. A study reported at the 2003 conference of the International Simulation and Game Association polled fifth graders to name their favorite video games. Of the 41 top titles, 85 percent contained violent content.

Turning violence into a part of everyday life, or even enjoyment, has a negative effect on a society. People feel less surprised and outraged when acts of brutality occur in real life. This desensitization may make people less likely to take a stand when they experience a violation of their own rights or see someone else's rights violated.

See also: Communities and Violence; Drugs and Violence; Media and Violence; School Violence; Teens and Violence

FURTHER READING

Langone, John. *Violence! Our Fastest-Growing Health Problem.* Boston: Little, Brown,1984.

Lawrence, Bruce, and Aisha Karim. *On Violence: A Reader.* Durham, N.C.: Duke University Press, 2008.

■ WAR

Large-scale organized violence between nations or ethnic groups. Reasons for armed conflict can include political disputes between nations, conflicts between political ideologies, racial or ethnic competition, and religious differences. The United Nations defines a "major war" as a military conflict that inflicts more than 1,000 battlefield casualties per year. According to the UN in 2009, there are 10 major wars and 32 civil, or "intrastate," wars with mostly civilian casualties, going on around the world. According to the Canadian organization Project Ploughshares, there are currently 28 "armed conflicts" in the world, spanning 24 countries. Additionally, the UN in 2009 maintains 18 peacekeeping missions around the world.

In almost every country, citizens support a military force. In some cases, that force is small and so is the percentage of the national budget devoted to military affairs. Other countries have huge military establishments costing billions of dollars and consuming a significant percentage of national resources. The costs of war quickly move beyond the money needed to pay soldiers, buy guns to put in their hands, and purchase ammunition for those weapons.

Q & A

Question: My brother signed up with the army to get help going to college. Now he's off in the middle of nowhere with a rifle! What can my family do?

Answer: Unfortunately, your brother is learning the difference between a peacetime and wartime army. In the 1990s, many people joined the military for job training or educational benefits. However, the basic job of any military organization is to fight. Your brother may face some difficult, even dangerous times during his tour of duty. It will be up to you and your family to maintain his morale with plenty of letters, messages, and packages from home.

FINANCIAL COSTS OF WAR

War is expensive. War-making involves much more than just the frontline troops, tanks, artillery pieces, and aircraft.

Military action requires transportation to get supplies and reinforcements to the war zone. Military organizations must also provide facilities for existing troops, maintenance shops to repair trucks and tanks, warehouses for equipment and spare parts, and much, much more. World War I cost the United States alone $22.6 billion. The expenses for all of the countries involved in the conflict cost nearly $200 trillion. In 2008, *The Washington Post* stated that the Iraq War would cost an estimated $3 trillion.

The book *War Finance* describes three ways to pay for armed conflict. The first involves going into debt. A country decides to worry about paying for the war after it is over and borrows money to pay for the extra expenses. The second method is taxation—the government requires that people pay more taxes and spends the extra money on the military. A third method is seigniorage. It is the profit a government can make between the actual cost of making a coin and its face value. If it costs the government 10 cents to make a quarter, but consumers value it at 25 cents, the government makes 15 cents on every coin.

The U.S. Civil War (1861–64) presents an illuminating look at war finance. The northern states raised money through borrowing and taxation. Congress raised existing taxes or instituted new taxes on all sorts of products. In 1861, the United States also introduced its first income tax. The South tried to borrow money to pay for war costs. When it could not borrow enough money, the Confederacy turned to its printing presses, simply producing paper money to pay its bills. Unfortunately, such money is subject to *inflation,* a decrease in the money's purchasing power as prices continually rise. By the war's end, Confederate money had suffered a 9,000 percent loss in purchasing power.

ENVIRONMENTAL COSTS

An article appearing in 2000 in the *Canadian Medical Association Journal* discussed the effects of war on health and the environment. The author suggested that military actions may exert four long-term effects on societies worldwide.

First, nuclear weapons have the capacity to destroy civilization and perhaps life on earth. Even if those weapons are never used, making and testing them creates **radioactive** waste that endangers living things, including humans.

The second area of concern comes from conventional bombing. Bombing destroys the infrastructure of a city—the built-in systems that allow people to live, work, and travel, among other things.

The third area of concern focuses on the effects of land mines. The International Committee for the Red Cross estimates that between 100 and 120 million of these have been buried in nations around the world over the last 60 years. Many of these relics from old wars are still active. The Federation of American Scientists Web site estimates that 26,000 people a year—500 a week—are killed or wounded by land mines. Land mines may be set off by farming or by children playing in an open field.

Finally, many military organizations intentionally destroy plant life and trees in war zones. Doing so diminishes the enemy's ability to secure food and deprives enemy soldiers of places to hide. The practice can also cause famine and starvation among the civilian population and often takes years to reverse.

COSTS TO THE FAMILY AND SOCIAL STRUCTURE

War also has an impact on civilians, including young children. Magne Raundalen, an internationally respected psychologist who specializes in treating children damaged by war or terror, was interviewed on Australian radio about the effects of the latest fighting on Iraqi children.

Raundalen maintained that these young people have three concerns about living in a war zone. They might be killed. They might be left alone after losing other members of their family. Finally, they are fearful about the future—what will be left for them after the war is over. Exposure to the ugliness of war leaves most children with emotional health issues that are likely to last a lifetime. Some have to deal with anxiety disorders—persistent, disturbing fears and possible flashbacks to terrifying wartime moments.

Since the mid-1990s, Dutch researchers have studied the impact of war on the ability of civilians to trust and have positive social relationships. Work with civilians who survived World War II showed that memories of wartime incidents remained years after the war ended, affecting sleep patterns and making it hard for some people to be optimistic about the future. Witnessing wartime violence and living through it destroys trust and optimism. Victims often lack a sense of security.

COSTS IN HUMAN LIFE

Perhaps the highest cost of war is counted in human lives. According to the U.S. Department of Defense, the Vietnam War took the lives of nearly 60,000 American servicemen and women. Nearly 20 years after the conflict, the Vietnamese government released figures that 1.1 million military people and 4 million civilians died during the war.

Before the 20th century, military planners concentrated on destroying the enemy's armed forces. However, the concept of total war has turned many civilians into targets. The *Encyclopaedia Britannica* estimated casualties for World War I at 8.5 million soldiers. However, 13 million civilians also died in that war. Casualty estimates for World War II ran even higher, with many sources quoting 50 million or more. The statistics quoted by the *Encyclopaedia Britannica* add up to 19,420,000 military deaths on both sides, with an additional 27,420,000 civilians, leaving a casualty total of almost 48 million. If those figures seem frightening, consider this—they do *not* include the vast numbers of people who were wounded, crippled, or blinded by that war.

TERRORIST ACTS

Many conflicts in the 20th century involved acts of terrorism. Terrorists are people who use violence as a weapon—to instill fear, influence political action, and promote a political or religious cause. Their focus is not an opposing army but a civilian population.

Between 1991 and 1995, a three-way struggle between the major ethnic groups in the former country of Yugoslavia took 250,000 lives. Militias formed by some ethnic groups in that struggle used rape and murder to drive other ethnic groups from their homes—an ugly process known as "ethnic cleansing."

In Rwanda, an African nation, terrorist acts by the Hutu tribe resulted in the murders of 800,000 members of the rival group, the Tutsis, within just three months. Many women were raped and mutilated before being murdered. Special efforts were made to eliminate anyone who might testify about the slaughter. In other parts of the world, conflicts may not reach such bloody levels, but the killing goes on for decades.

The use of terrorism allows a small number of people to have a huge impact. Counterterrorism expert Gayle Rivers explains the effect very simply in his book, *The War Against the Terrorists:* "Kill one, frighten a million."

Terrorists seek out civilian targets, not only because it is easier to attack unarmed civilians than soldiers, but also because a well-placed bomb in a shopping mall guarantees publicity for the terrorists and their cause.

Consider the grim mathematics of September 11, 2001. At the cost of the lives of 19 terrorists, Al Qaeda destroyed the World Trade Center and damaged the Pentagon, the military headquarters of the United States. The attacks killed more than 3,000 people and generated weeks of media coverage. On September 10, 2001, few people knew anything about Al Qaeda. After September 11, no one could pick up a newspaper or turn on a television or radio without hearing about the group.

Fact Or Fiction?

Violence never solves anything.

The Facts: Looking back at history, one might discover that violence has solved a number of things. For instance, the Revolutionary War determined whether Americans would remain British colonists or become citizens of a nation of their own. The Civil War solved the problem of slavery. World War II removed the Nazis from power, freed countries around the world from dictatorships, and ended Japanese military ambitions. Fifty years of military preparedness and resistance also ended the threat of Communism. Studies of history also show that solving one problem is no guarantee of living "happily ever after"—new problems keep developing.

THE CHANGING NATURE OF WAR

Wars are changing. Today few wars involve only military targets. Civilians are increasingly involved. Their involvements raises the costs of war immeasurably.

See also: Community and Violence; Weapons of Violence

FURTHER READING

Brownlie, Alison. *Why Do People Fight Wars?* Austin, Tex.: Raintree/ Steck-Vaugh, 2002.

Kaldor, Mary. *New and Old Wars: Organized Violence in a Global Era.* Palo Alto, Calif.: Stanford University Press, 2007.

Ward, Geoffrey C., and Ken Burns. *The War: An Intimate History, 1941–1945.* New York: Knopf, 2007.

■ WEAPONS OF VIOLENCE

Instruments that can be used for offense or defense in combat. Conventional weapons may fire projectiles, like bullets or cannon balls, or have sharp edges that cut. However, many seemingly harmless objects can be turned into weapons, like baseball bats, pieces of pipe, or even broken glass bottles.

GUNS

Guns have long been a part of American life, from the Kentucky long rifle to the Colt six-shooter. Americans own weapons for many reasons. Some keep a gun in their homes for protection. Others use them for hunting and sport shooting. Still others use guns to intimidate or bully.

According to a 2009 fact sheet produced by the Brady Campaign to Prevent Gun Violence, more than 100,000 people were shot. Approximately 30,896 died from gun violence, while an estimated 69,863 people survived. Some 3,218 children and adolescents between

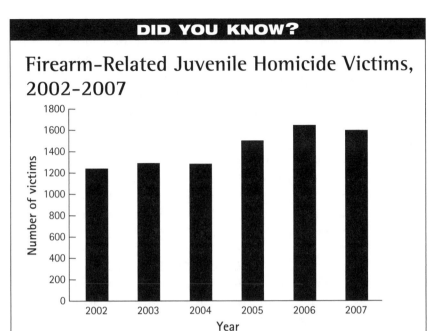

DID YOU KNOW?

Firearm-Related Juvenile Homicide Victims, 2002-2007

The number of juvenile homicide victims who were killed with guns was relatively unchanged until 2005, the year in which the number spiked. Fortunately, the numbers are now starting to come down.

Source: Adopted from the *Sourcebook of Criminal Justice Statistics Online, 2007.* Bureau of Justice Statistics. Accessed 05/20/09.

birth and age 19 died from gun violence. Another 17,566 were shot and survived.

Laurence Steinberg, a psychologist specializing in adolescent development, observed, "What is different about youth violence in America is not that the violence our young people commit is more frequent, but that it is more lethal, and this is because of the weapons they use."

Young people in the United States have access to guns at an earlier and earlier age. The Centers for Disease Control and Prevention (CDC) conduct an assessment of adolescents every two years. The CDC's Youth Risk Behavior Surveillance System (YRBSS) asks several violence-related questions. In the 2007 survey, the CDC learned that about 5.2 percent of all students had carried a gun on at least one of the 30 days preceding the survey. According to the National Center for Injury Prevention and Control, homicide ranks as the second-leading killer of 15- to 24-year-olds and the fourth-leading killer for the 10–14 and 24–35 age group. The majority of these homicides are from gun injuries. According to a 2007 report by the National Center for Education Statistics and the Bureau of Justice Statistics, 6 percent of students in grades nine through 12 admitted to bringing a weapon to school within the past month.

According to the Bureau of Justice Statistics, in 2006, 55 percent of all homicides were committed with a handgun. Another 16 percent were committed using other types of firearms. According to the National Crime Victimization Survey for 2006, 21.7 percent of robberies were committed with a gun. Guns were involved in assaults 6.6 percent of the time.

PHYSICAL FIGHTS

Fists, feet, and nails can also be used as weapons. High school students reported in the 2007 YRBSS that 35.5 percent had been in a physical fight during the previous year. More than 44 percent of the boys and 25 percent of girls reported fighting in the previous year at least one time. More than 4 percent of these students were hurt badly enough to seek medical attention after the fight.

A number of schools have set out to teach students that violence is not the only response to conflict. Violence prevention programs include the development of skills in anger management, conflict resolution, problem solving, and stress management. When students possess these skills, they are more likely to avoid violence.

CUTTING OBJECTS

Knives and other sharp objects can also serve as weapons. According to the Bureau of Justice Statistics, knives and other sharp objects played a part in 6.2 percent of all violent crime in 2006. That year, 5,685,620 violent crimes took place in the United States, which means that knives figured in approximately 352,000 of those crimes. Blade weapons were used in 190,171 robberies, 326,627 aggravated assaults (assaults where the attacker used a weapon), and 18,683 rapes or sexual assaults.

Many people who might find it difficult to get a gun can easily buy a knife. Box cutters, for instance, are used in most stores to unpack merchandise. The cutter retracts into the handle, so it's convenient. One can carry it in a pocket. The tool is inexpensive and readily available. Some cities have tried to ban the sale of box cutters to people under the age of 18. A 1999 New York City press release described an undercover sting operation in which teens went into stores to buy box cutters. Of the 52 shops tested, 25 percent sold this potential weapon. Two years later, terrorist hijackers carried box cutters on at least one of the planes used in the attacks on September 11, 2001.

FIRES AND BOMBS

Arson is a crime; it is the intentional, malicious burning of a building. The National Fire Protection Association (NFPA) reported 323,200 intentional fires in 2006. In 2007 fires were responsible for 305 deaths and caused $733 million in damages. Law enforcement officials have a difficult time finding those responsible for arson. In 2007, only 18 percent of all arsons resulted in an arrest. Fifty-two percent of those arrested were under the age of 18. In fact, the NFPA says that juveniles make up the highest percentage of arsonists. Over half of all arson crimes are committed by youths under the age 18, with 2.8 percent under the age of 15, and 3 percent under the age of 10.

Fire also results from the use of bombs, especially in a military situation. By the end of 2003, some 35 military conflicts around the world provided ample opportunity for the use of explosives, whether fired from artillery pieces or dropped from airplanes.

Advancements in technology have considerably improved airplane bombing runs. So-called **smart bombs** incorporate video cameras and guidance systems. Using information relayed back to the bomber, personnel aboard the airplane can direct the bomb's course, much as people control movement on a video game screen.

Fact Or Fiction?

If some country starts making nukes, we ought to go in there and stop them.

The Facts: Some countries have moved to stop others from trying to develop nuclear weapons, usually by intercepting scientific equipment before it reaches the nuclear researchers. In 1981, Israeli warplanes attacked and destroyed the Osirak nuclear facility in Iraq, destroying it. At the time, Iraq was believed to be within years of creating a nuclear bomb.

Unfortunately, it is often difficult to tell exactly how far a nation has come along the road to nuclear capability. In 1998, India detonated three nuclear bombs, surprising the world and U.S. intelligence agencies. Even through the country was under the surveillance of spy satellites, intelligence analysts did not detect the preparations for the underground tests.

As one of the Indian nuclear researchers put it in a 1998 *National Review* article, "It's a matter on their intelligence being good, our deception being better."

The most powerful weapon today is the nuclear bomb. Only a few countries have developed nuclear capability, but the fact that a number of nations are trying to build these weapons is of grave concern to military and political leaders worldwide. Nuclear bombs achieve their destructive power by forcing atoms to split, releasing tremendous amounts of energy. From the 1950s through the 1980s, the cold war—the political and military conflict between the United States and the former Soviet Union—spurred the creation of huge nuclear arsenals. Many people believed the world would soon be destroyed. The missiles were never used. Today, many fear that the technology for creating those nuclear weapons will fall into the hands of terrorists.

Nuclear bombs saw combat action only at the end of World War II. In 1944, the United States became the only nation to ever use nuclear weapons in combat. The nation dropped two atom bombs on Japan: one on Hiroshima and one on Nagasaki. The toll was devastating. Over 200,000 people were killed. When a nuclear bomb explodes, it immediately creates an intense, incomparable surge of heat that reaches 300 million degrees centigrade at its core. When these bombs were dropped, the top of the cloud formed by the blast reached 17,000 feet. Everyone within 1,000 yards of the blast died, and people as far away as two miles needed significant medical attention for radiation burns. Buildings were immediately consumed in the blast. In total, the first atom bomb killed between 30 and 40 percent of the population of Hiroshima.

The tragedy does not end there, however. A nuclear explosion produces more than heat. It creates debris that radiates nuclear particles and energy waves. These **radioactive** by-products are extremely harmful to living things. Radioactive fallout stays in the air and collects on the ground, causing many health problems for people in the area. In the months after the Hiroshima bombing, residents developed massive scar tissue from burns, cataracts, leukemia and other cancers, hair loss, birth defects, and infertility. It may be another hundred years before we know the true long-term consequences.

CHEMICAL AND BIOLOGICAL WEAPONS

Chemical weapons are devices designed to cause death or other harm through the poisonous properties of chemicals. **Biological weapons** use disease-causing organisms like bacteria or viruses, or toxins (poisons) found in nature to kill or incapacitate people. Along with nuclear weapons, these devices are called **weapons of mass destruction** because of the dangers they pose. These weapons can destroy the lives of thousands, even millions of people.

Chemical warfare was introduced during World War I with the use of poison gas. More recently these weapons have been associated with terrorists. In 1995, Japanese cult members released sarin in the Tokyo subway. Sarin is a **nerve gas,** a chemical agent that attacks the human nervous system. The poison gas was released in several places in the subway system, killing 11 and injuring 5,500 people.

In 2001, during the weeks after September 11, letters containing spores of anthrax, a deadly disease, were sent to five media offices and two U.S. senators. As a result of their exposure to the disease, 22 people were infected with anthrax, and five died of inhalation anthrax. Two of the fatalities occurred after anthrax powder contaminated the mail as it was being processed at a postal facility.

During the dictatorship of Saddam Hussein, Iraq developed an arsenal of chemical weapons that were used during the Iran-Iraq War and to put down internal rebellions. Concern that Iraq was developing new and more dangerous weapons of mass destruction was a major rationale for the American-led invasion that deposed Saddam Hussein. Since 2003, there have been more than 500 chemical weapons found in Iraq.

Weapons were probably among the earliest tools developed by humankind. Science and technology have allowed the production of increasingly sophisticated weapons. One fact remains, however. Whether it is a complicated virus developed in a laboratory or an improvised club snatched up from the street, weapons can—and often do—kill.

See also: Criminals and Violent Activity; Drugs and Violence; Teens and Violence; War

FURTHER READING
Guy, John. *Weapons and Warfare*. New York: Barrons, 1998.
Kahaner, Larry. *AK-47: The Weapon That Changed the Face of War*. Hoboken, N.J.: Wiley, 2007.

■ WORKPLACE VIOLENCE

A variety of aggressive and harmful behaviors that take place in factories, offices, and other places of business. At times, workplace violence has featured prominently in the news, as the following stories suggest. In March 2008, four men were killed in Santa Maria, California, while working at their junkyard. In April 2008, a man shot his coworker and then committed suicide in Randolf, Massachusetts. In May 2009, an incident occurred in which a man killed his boss and a coworker.

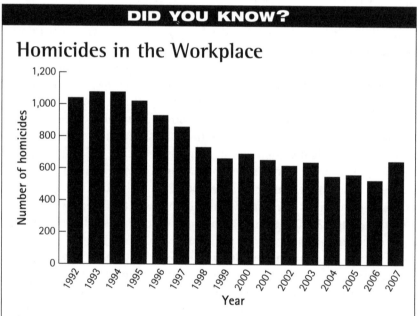

DID YOU KNOW?

Homicides in the Workplace

According to the government report published in 2005, since 1994, workplace homicides have been steadily decreasing, with the exception of slight increases in 2000, 2003, and 2007.

Source: *The Editor's Desk: Workplace Homicides Decline in 2004*. Bureau of Labor Statistics, 2007.

According to the U.S. Department of Labor Bureau Statistics, in 2006, there were 540 incidents of workplace homicide. Contrary to what the media reports, most of these incidents were not committed by workers. Robbers and other perpetrators committed 371 homicides, while coworkers committed 70 homicides. Clients or customers accounted for 53 homicides; relatives committed 21 homicides; and other acquaintances committed 25 homicides.

When the media discusses workplace violence, it usually concentrates on murder and **sexual harassment**—unwelcome sexual advances, requests for sexual favors, or other verbal or physical conduct of a sexual nature that are made conditions of employment, used as a basis for employment decisions or create a work environment that interferes with job performance. Less newsworthy but still dangerous situations include threats from angry customers and patrons, worker/management disputes, and abusive initiation rites for new employees.

Regardless of the type of violence people encounter at work, common threads connect these incidents. An article in the *Journal of Occupational and Environmental Medicine* discussed common factors related to workplace violence. Work environments with high levels of stress can lead to violence. When plants close or companies engage in downsizing, reducing the number of employees, violence may also result. Workplaces that condone on-the-job bullying may foster confrontations when those who have been bullied become so stressed that they resort to violence. People with jobs in health care, social services, and other industries that deal directly with the public may also encounter violence in the workplace.

HAZING IN THE WORKPLACE

Hazing is a form of initiation. New members of an organization are required to perform humiliating tasks or face rough practical jokes as a condition of employment. Sometimes workplace hazing is just silly, like having "the new kid" look for forms that don't exist or asking a new worker to pick up a tool that has been welded to the floor. However, these rites can isolate new workers, with veterans treating them like second-class citizens, verbally harassing them, and even interfering with their work.

The employee-rights organization Job Watch reports that hazing activities often escalate. The longer rituals are allowed to continue, the more extreme they can become. Some workers simply can't handle the abuse physically or emotionally. Employees may become depressed, experience a lack of desire to return to work, or be generally unproductive at work. Some people have more extreme reactions, resulting in shooting incidents much like the ones in high schools where victims of bullying lash out at those abusing them.

UNIONS AND ANGER

In many industries, workers have joined labor unions to protect their rights, improve working conditions, and seek higher compensation. When negotiations between labor and management fail to resolve a conflict, the union may call a **strike**, or work stoppage. The United States has a more violent history of labor relations compared to many other industrial nations. As the book *The War on Labor and the Left* points out, 700 American strikers were killed in labor disputes between 1877 and 1968. In Britain, only one striker has been killed since 1911.

Strikes are often emotional times, with feelings running high between those who have walked off the job and those who refuse to honor picket lines. Even old friends can find themselves on opposite sides. Since President Ronald Reagan replaced nearly all of the country's air traffic controllers after a strike in the 1980s, more and more employers have chosen to bring in what they call "replacement workers" when unions attempt to shut down workplaces. Union members see these workers as "strikebreakers" and "scabs."

The use of replacement workers has resulted in longer strikes, greater hardship for strikers, anger, and violence. The National Institute for Labor Relations Research, a pro-management organization, identified 8,799 incidents of labor union violence in the news between 1975 and 1998. The organization has also complained of a "loophole" created by the U.S. Supreme Court in laws to control labor unions. When striking electricians were accused of sabotaging company equipment, the Court ruled that the action was fair, because workers were trying to advance their union's legitimate objectives.

Based on this decision, only 258 convictions have resulted from the 8,799 accusations over the past 23 years. Replacement workers and those who chose not to participate in strikes have faced verbal threats and harassment, physical attacks, and even murder.

RESPONSES TO HARASSMENT

Sexual harassment has become a growing problem over the last 60 years, as more and more women have entered the workforce.

Harassment includes unwanted touching or grabbing, sexual advances, requests for sexual favors, sexual jokes, or constant pestering for a date. Turning down these advances often has a negative impact on a person's chances for promotion or pay increases.

Q & A

Question: If I meet someone I like at work, do sexual harassment laws prohibit me from asking him/her out on a date?

Answer: Technically, no, although for many reasons it is not advised you date a coworker. Harassment has to do with the creation of a threatening, intimidating, or hostile work environment. If you ask, and the person says no, then you have to let it go. If you keep asking, then you cross a line. If turning you down means that the individual will be punished in some way at work, then you have also crossed the line.

In formerly all-male work environments, crude jokes, offensive language, macho horseplay, and posting pinups or centerfolds were tolerated and even accepted. These behaviors and many others are not appropriate in mixed company. By the 1960s, those behaviors were not only offensive, but also illegal. Lawsuits based on Title VII of the Civil Rights Act of 1964 forced many companies to make changes in the workplace.

Through the 1980s and 1990s, many companies began to establish rules of behavior. The penalties for violating these rules often began with a warning but could lead to dismissal if the behavior and the attitudes that prompted that behavior did not change. The law emphasized the dangers of creating "a hostile work environment."

One of the best ways to prevent harassment is to improve one's communication skills. Men and women are socialized differently in the United States, making it easy for someone to say or do the wrong thing at the wrong time. If someone has said something that offends a coworker, immediate communication can minimize the damage. The person who is offended should explain why the remark or action was distasteful, and the offender should apologize.

Fact Or Fiction?

Workplace shootings are the most common form of workplace violence.

The Facts: Murder at work makes up a very small percentage of workplace violence. In fact, only one out of every 2,000 acts of workplace violence results in death. It seems high because the murders are the only part of workplace violence the media covers. Almost 400,000 aggravated assaults (assaults with a weapon) occur each year at work, most of those as a carryover from domestic violence incidents. More than half of all violent incidents are threats of physical harm, harassment, or other acts which create an unhealthy environment to work in.

WORKPLACE VIOLENCE PREVENTION

In response to the problems associated with workplace violence, many organizations and consultants have developed programs to protect employees. The National Institute for Occupational Safety and Health provides workplace violence-prevention strategies for companies to follow. Company-specific policies need to be written and shared with all employees. Employees also need to be trained in violence-prevention strategies.

Organized teams examine the company's business facilities to assess the vulnerability of employees to four kinds of violence—from strangers, clients or customers, coworkers, and personal relationships. A workplace violence program must also address security issues. Do people work alone? Are they responsible for valuable items? Are staffing levels appropriate? Do workers have training to anticipate problems and control them? Does the company's written violence prevention policies treat all employees fairly? Have they been trained to resolve conflicts and disputes? Does the program allow employees to restrict access by family members? Do supervisors have training to deal with family violence issues and keep the situation confidential?

The U.S. Office of Personnel Management also maintains information on workplace violence prevention. These are indicators that may help to identify potentially dangerous workers:

- Direct or veiled threats of harm
- Intimidating, belligerent, harassing, bullying, or other inappropriate and aggressive behavior

- Numerous conflicts with supervisors and other employees
- Bringing a weapon to the workplace, brandishing a weapon in the workplace, making inappropriate references to guns, or showing a fascination with weapons
- Statements showing fascination with incidents of workplace violence, statements indicating approval of the use of violence to resolve a problem, or statements indicating identification with perpetrators of workplace homicides
- Statements indicating desperation (over family, financial, and other personal problems) to the point of contemplating suicide
- Drug/alcohol abuse
- Extreme changes in behaviors.

While the guidelines warn that participants in the program must avoid **profiling**–judging individuals by stereotypes–the behaviors listed cannot be ignored.

Americans work hard. Worrying about harassment or violence at work makes a tough job even tougher. Awareness of the kinds of problems one can face plus proper training to deal with them can go a long way toward avoiding workplace violence.

See also: Assault and Bullying; School Violence; Sexual Violence

FURTHER READING
Chaiet, Donna. *Staying Safe at Work.* New York: Rosen Publishing Group, 1995.
Paludi, Michele, Rudy V. Nydegger, and Carmen A. Paludi. *Understanding Workplace Violence: A Guide for Managers and Employees.* Westport, Conn.: Praeger Publishers, 2006.

HOTLINES AND HELP SITES

D.A.R.E. (Drug Abuse Resistance Education) America
URL: http://www.dare.com
Phone: 1-800-223-DARE (3273)
Mission: Founded in 1983 in Los Angeles, D.A.R.E. has proven so successful that it is now being implemented in nearly 80 percent of our nation's school districts and in more than 54 countries around the world. This year 36 million school children around the world—26 million in the United States—will benefit from D.A.R.E., which gives kids the skills they need to avoid involvement in drugs, gangs, and violence.
Programs: A police officer–led series of classroom lessons that teaches children from kindergarten through 12th grade how to resist peer pressure and live productive drug- and violence-free lives

Division of Violence Prevention, National Center for Injury Prevention and Control (NCIPC), Centers for Disease Control and Prevention (CDC)
URL: http://www.cdc.gov/ncipc
Phone: 1-800-232-4636
Mission: The CDC provides credible information to enhance health decisions and promotes health through strong partnerships. The NCIPC focuses on helping people avoid injuries, both unintentional and intentional.
Programs: The Division of Violence Prevention has represented the CDC's focus on violence prevention since the early 1980s, when efforts included the prevention of youth violence, suicide, and

suicide attempts. The division offers information in the areas of child maltreatment, intimate partner violence, sexual violence, suicide, and youth violence.

G.R.E.A.T. (Gang Resistance Education and Training)
URL: http://www.great-online.org
Phone: 1-800-726-7070
Mission: Designed to help children set goals for themselves, resist pressures, learn how to resolve conflicts without violence, and understand how gangs and youth violence impact the quality of their lives
Programs: A school-based program developed by the Bureau of Alcohol, Tobacco, Firearms, and Explosives and other federal law enforcement agencies. G.R.E.A.T. students discover for themselves the ramifications of gang and youth violence through structured exercises and interactive approaches to learning. The program provides training and a classroom curriculum.

National Center for Victims of Crime
URL: http://www.ncvc.org
Phone: 202-467-8700
National helpline: 1-800-FYI-CALL (394-2255)
Mission: To forge a national commitment to help victims of crime rebuild their lives. Dedicated to serving individuals, families, and communities harmed by crime
Programs: Since 1985, the organization has worked with more than 10,000 grassroots organizations and criminal justice agencies serving millions of crime victims. It offers supportive counseling, practical information about crime and victimization, referrals to local community resources, as well as skilled advocacy in the criminal justice and social service systems.

National Domestic Violence Hotline
URL: http://www.ndvh.org
Phone: 1-800-799-SAFE (7233)
Mission: To answer phone calls from victims of domestic violence, family members, and friends from all over the world for crisis intervention, referrals, and general information about domestic violence
Programs: With a database of more than 4,000 shelters and service providers across the United States, Puerto Rico, Alaska, Hawaii,

and the U.S. Virgin Islands, the hotline provides callers with information they might otherwise have found difficult or impossible to obtain. The hotline is available 24 hours a day, 365 days a year.

National Hopeline Network: Kristin Brooks Hope Center
URL: http://www.hopeline.com
Phone: 540-338-5756
Hotline: 1-800-SUICIDE (784-2433)
Mission: A nonprofit organization dedicated to suicide prevention, intervention, and healing, by providing a single point of entry to community-based crisis services through telephone and Internet-based technologies; by bringing national attention and access to services for postpartum depression and other women's mood disorders; through education and advocacy; through formal research and evaluation of crisis line services; and by championing the need for national funding for community-based suicide prevention crisis services.
Programs: Connects callers to a certified crisis center nearest the caller's location; services are available 24 hours a day, seven days a week.

National Institute on Alcohol Abuse and Alcoholism (NIAAA)
URL: http://www.niaaa.nih.gov
Mission: Provides leadership in the national effort to reduce alcohol-related problems
Programs: Conducts and supports research in a wide range of scientific areas, including genetics, neuroscience, epidemiology, health risks and benefits of alcohol consumption, prevention, and treatment; translates and disseminates research findings to health-care providers, researchers, policy makers, and the public

National Institute on Drug Abuse (NIDA)
URL: http://www.nida.nih.gov
Mission: To lead the nation in bringing the power of science to bear on drug abuse and addiction
Programs: Furthers understanding of how drugs of abuse affect the brain and behavior and ensures the rapid and effective transfer of scientific data to policy makers, drug abuse practitioners, other health-care practitioners, and the general public

National Institute on Media and the Family
Phone: 1-888-672-5437
URL: http://www.mediafamily.org

Mission: Founded by David Walsh, Ph.D., in 1996, this organization examines the impact of electronic media on families, working to help parents and communities monitor what their kids watch

Programs: Provides information about the impact of media on children and gives people who care about children the resources they need to make informed choices

Rape, Abuse & Incest National Network (RAINN)

URL: http://www.rainn.org

Hotline: 1-800-656-HOPE (4673)

Mission: To serve as the nation's largest anti–sexual assault organization

Programs: Offers counseling resources, prevention tips, and news; operates the National Sexual Assault Hotline; and carries out programs to prevent sexual assault, help victims, and ensure that rapists are brought to justice

GLOSSARY

abandonment   to leave or desert a person, especially a person who cannot survive without help

addiction   the state of becoming physically or psychologically dependent on a drug

aggravated assault   a legal term referring to an attack made on a person, usually with a weapon, with the intention of causing serious harm

autonomic nervous system   the part of the nervous system which controls involuntary body actions, such as the beating of the heart

autonomy-oriented   a psychological classification under self-determination theory, describing those who believe their responses and actions come from within themselves

behavior modification   a form of psychological treatment aimed at changing or stopping a destructive or unwanted behavior

Benzedrine   a trademarked name for an amphetamine drug, which acts as a stimulant, speeding up the nervous system and body functions

biological weapons   weapons using disease-causing organisms or poisonous by-products from these organisms to destroy life

cannabis   *See* marijuana.

castration the process of removing or depriving the use of the sexual organs

chemical weapons weapons using the poisonous effects of chemical compounds to incapacitate or kill people

chronic long-lasting or repeated; used to describe any illness that is not easily cured

chronic community violence a situation where residents in a locality experience frequent and prolonged exposure to weapons, crime, and random acts of violence

cocaine an addictive stimulant drug that speeds up the nervous system and body functions

cognitive behavioral treatment psychological therapy where patients work to understand the thoughts and emotions behind their behavior

community policing policy initiatives to create a partnership between police and communities in preventing crime

community service an alternative to a prison sentence whereby convicted criminal offenders undertake some effort to help the district or locality where they live

conflict resolution the settlement of personal differences between people by means of effective communication, often guided by a mediator

control-oriented a psychological classification under self-determination theory, describing those who believe their behavior is the result of external actions and influences

court costs the expenses involved in administering a legal trial

crack a very powerful, inexpensive form of cocaine

criminal homicide the unlawful taking of a human life, including murder and manslaughter

cycle of events in cognitive-behavioral psychological therapy, the chain of thoughts and incidents that leads up to an action

depressant a drug which depresses, or slows down, the nervous system and body functions

depression a psychological state distinguished by feelings of sadness, low self-worth, and a lack of energy

discipline punishment, especially that which aims to produce improved moral behavior

domestic violence physical or sexual violence or psychological abuse committed by family members or intimate partners

drive-by shooting a form of intergang violence where groups of gang members in the street are fired upon by rival gang members in a passing car

drug rehabilitation the process by which an addict overcomes dependency on a drug

elder abuse violence expressed against a person 60 years or older, including physical, sexual, and emotional abuse, financial exploitation, abandonment, and neglect

eldercide the murder of an older person, age 65 or older

emotional abuse mistreatment by attacking a person's feelings through threats, humiliation, or other harmful actions

excusable homicide a legal situation where a death occurs as a result of a person's actions but without criminal intent

family breakdown a failing in the family structure where family members no longer feel an emotional connection

felonious homicide *See* criminal homicide.

felony   a classification of more serious crimes, punishable by harsher sentences

fighting words   forms of expression calculated to inflame listeners and incite violent actions

financial exploitation   misusing money or financial resources of persons one is supposed to be caring for

fundamentalism   rigid religious belief in a set of principles or an inspired religious text

gatekeeper   in suicide prevention programs, a person trained to recognize the warning signs of suicide in individuals and who picks such people out of groups, referring them for help

gene   a structure that transmits characteristics and functions between generations of living things

genocide   the systematic, planned extermination of a racial or cultural group

group therapy   a form of psychological treatment involving interaction between more than one patient

guided self-help program   a form of self-improvement undertaken with information and advice from a therapist, book, computer program, or the like

hallucinogen   a drug which causes false perceptions of reality for users

hardy personality   a psychological classification of people who can successfully handle stress

hazing   a form of initiation for new members of a group, usually involving the accomplishment of difficult or humiliating tasks or undergoing practical jokes

hormone   a body chemical which affects various organs, initiating, stopping, or modifying its function

individual self-help   a form of dealing with problems by working on them alone and by helping others, as occurs in recovery groups like Alcoholics Anonymous

infanticide   taking the life of a child less than five years old

inhalants   intoxicating substances which cause dizziness and other effects by being breathed in, such as aerosol fumes

intimate partner abuse   acts of verbal or physical violence against a spouse, a live-in lover, or between people who are dating

intravenous   into or involving the veins, as in the term intravenous drug abuse, where substances are injected into the body through the veins

juvenile court   a legal system devised to deal with criminal behavior by young people, with the aim of helping them develop into useful members of society

laws   the body of rules governing the affairs of a community, state, or nation

mandatory sentencing laws   legal articles setting forth strict guidelines for federal judges in sentencing convicted offenders

manslaughter   the taking of human life without the intention of doing injury

marijuana   an intoxicating plant which, when smoked, causes feelings of euphoria—great happiness—in users

methamphetamines   an addictive stimulant drug that speeds up the nervous system and body functions

misdemeanor   a legal classification of less serious crimes, punished with a fine or a brief prison sentence

murder   the intentional taking of a human life

narcotics   drugs that dull the senses, bring on sleep, and, with continued use, result in addiction

negative reinforcement   a psychological term for a punishment or unwelcome result coming from a particular behavior

neglect   failure to provide for a child's or adult's basic needs; can be emotional, psychological, or physical

nerve gas   a chemical weapon which attacks the function of the nerves, thereby paralyzing the muscles they control

neurotransmitters   body chemicals which transmit information from one nerve cell to another

overdose   taking an excessive or fatal dose of a drug

parole   the release of a prisoner before his or her sentence is over, on the condition of the person's good behavior

peer mediation   a method of resolving conflicts where both of the arguing sides work with an equal in their community to develop a compromise

physical abuse   inflicting pain or physical harm on a person

positive reinforcement   a psychological term for a reward of desired result coming from a particular behavior

prejudice   a judgment about people or things formed in advance, without examining the facts

probation   the action of suspending a legal sentence and granting freedom to a convicted offender on the promise of good behavior

profiling   the process of developing a list of characteristics about a particular offender; also using lists of characteristics indiscriminately to identify whole classes of people as potential offenders

rape   sexual intercourse achieved against another person's will by force or the threat of force

recidivism   a tendency to fall back into former behavior, especially criminal habits

relapse prevention   a form of psychological therapy aimed at keeping people from falling back into unwelcome forms of behavior

robbery   unlawfully taking the property of another through force or threat of force

schizophrenia   a mental disorder marked by loss of touch with reality

sedative   a drug with a calming, tranquilizing effect

self-determination theory   a psychological theory that views people's motives and personalities as expressions of free will

serotonin   a body chemical found mainly in the brain that is capable of raising body temperature, controlling certain types of muscles, and changing behavior

sexual abuse   forcing or tricking another person into unwanted sexual contact

sexual bribery   using a superior social or employment position to offer desirable consideration in return for sexual favors

sexual coercion   using a superior social or employment position to threaten a person into offering sexual favors

skinheads   followers of extreme political movements advocating racial superiority, so named because of the extremely short haircuts they favor

smart bomb   explosive weapons that can be dropped from airplanes and guided to targets

stereotype   an oversimplified and often inaccurate idea, opinion, or belief

steroid or 'roid rage   outbursts of anger caused by body chemistry imbalances due to the use of steroid drugs

stimulant   a drug which speeds up the nervous system and body functions

stressor   anything that causes stress

strike   a work stoppage by employees, especially employees organized in a union

terrorism   the use of violence and fear to achieve an end, especially a political end

three Cs of hardiness   commitment, challenge, and control; elements in creating a personality that will resist stress

token economy   an element of behavior modification that offers rewards for desired behavior

tolerance   the process by which a human body becomes accustomed to an addictive substance, requiring larger and larger doses to achieve a high

trigger   a psychological term for an event which stimulates anger and may provoke a violent response

truth-in-sentencing laws   legal controls ensuring that imprisoned offenders serve at least 85 percent of their sentences

turf   territory controlled by a gang

weapons of mass destruction   certain forms of arms—nuclear, biological, or chemical weapons—that can cause widespread damage either to property or to populations

withdrawal   the physical symptoms connected with ending the use of addictive drugs

INDEX

Boldface page numbers indicate extensive treatment of a topic.

A

AAP. *See* American Academy of Pediatrics (AAP) 43
abuse. *See* family violence
acquaintance rape 122–123
Administration on Children, Youth and Families 126
African Americans. *See* hate crimes; violence against populations
Aggression and Violent Behavior 40, 154
Aggressive Behavior 80
alcohol and violence **13–16**
  about 6, 8
  and cultural expectations 16
  effects of alcohol 13–14
  and family violence 44
  and hate crimes 62
  and personality 15
  and rehabilitation 130
  and teenage violence 142–143
  theories about 14–15
American Academy of Pediatrics (AAP) 43

American Foundation for Suicide Prevention 14
American Journal of Orthopsychiatry 79
American Journal of Preventative Medicine 128
American Journal of Psychiatry 77
American Journal of Sociology 95
American Medical Association 42
American Prosecutors Resource Institute 141
American Psychological Association (APA) 29–30, 68, 117
American Psychologist 27, 28
American Street Gang, The (Klein) 56, 59
anger management **17–22**
  and pain 21–22
  programs for 18–20
  and thinking errors 17–18
Annual Review of Public Health 91
anthrax 149–150
Anti-Defamation League 64
APA. *See* American Psychological Association (APA)
Archives of General Psychiatry 79, 151, 166
arson 179

Arts in Psychotherapy, The 100–101
assault and bullying 22–27
  dealing with 26–27
  definition of 4, 23–25
  effects of 25
  and suicide 143
  victims of 7, 139–140
Auburn Prison 70–72

B

Basic and Applied Social Psychology 103
behavior modification 96
Behavior Science and the Law 96, 98
Behavioural and Cognitive Psychotherapy 18
Behaviour Research and Therapy 79
Biological Psychiatry 83
biological weapons 181
bioterrorism 149–150
BJS (Bureau of Justice Statistics). *See* Bureau of Justice Statistics (BJS)
Black's Law Dictionary 66
bombs 179–181
Brady Campaign to Prevent Gun Violence 176–177
British Association of Social Workers 126
British Journal of Psychology 136
British Journal of Psychiatry, The 21
Building Coalitions 101 29
Bulletin of Clinical Psychopharmacology 80
bullying. *See* assault and bullying
Bureau of Justice Statistics (BJS)
  alcohol and violence 13
  costs of violence 127
  hate crimes 154, 157
  incarceration 32, 77
  law enforcement 33–34
  paroles 98
  recidivism 94–95
  sexual violence 119, 121

  victims of violence 138
  weapons of violence 178

C

Canadian Medical Association Journal 173
car accidents. *See* road rage
causes of violent behavior. *See* violent behavior, causes of
CCV. *See* chronic community violence (CCV)
CDC. *See* Centers for Disease Control and Prevention (CDC)
Center for the Study and Prevention of Violence 139
Centers for Disease Control and Prevention (CDC)
  costs of violence 127, 128
  homicide 66, 69
  prevention strategies 31
  school violence 109–110
  steroids 168
  suicide 132, 133
  teenage violence 138
  terrorism 149
  weapons of violence 177
chemical weapons 181
child abuse 41–42, 43, 125–126
Child Abuse & Neglect 105
Child Abuse Review 125
Child Adolescent Psychiatric Clinics of North America 162
Child Protection 41
chronic community violence (CCV) 27
Chronicle of the American Driver and Traffic Safety Education Association 106
City Journal 86
Clinton, William Jefferson 111
cognitive-behavioral therapy 96–98
Columbine High School 68, 91, 109

Committee on the Training Needs of Health Professionals 42
communication skills 114–116
communities and violence **27–31**
  neglecting reports of violence 28
  prevention strategies 29
  taking action 29–30
community service 35, 98–100
Comprehensive Community Reanimation Process 55
Comprehensive National Cybersecurity Initiative (CNCI) 149
conflict resolution 8, 60, 178
Corrections Management Quarterly 99
costs of violence. *See* social costs of violence; war
Crime & Justice 58
Crime Act 32
Crime Victimization 2003 127
Criminal Justice and Behavior 161
criminals and violent activity **31–35**
  laws 32–34
  legal definitions 31–32
  perpetrators of violence 7–9
  punishment 34–35
Criminology 34, 87, 95
Current Directions in Psychological Science 162
cyberterrorism 147–149
cycle of violence 100–106

D

Darfur 158
date rape 122–123
Date Rape Prevention Book (Lindquist) 123
dating violence 138–139
delinquents 35
Denning, Dorothy 147
depressants 37. *See also* alcohol and violence
depression 132–133, 134
Diallo, Amadou 86

discipline v. abuse 42–44
domestic violence. *See* family violence
Drinking Patterns and Their Consequences (Grant and Litvak) 16
drive-by shootings 53
driving. *See* road rage
drugs and violence **36–41**
  intravenous drug use 38
  loss of control 39–40
  steroids 167–170
  types of drugs 37–38

E

Eastern State Penitentiary 70
Education, U.S. Department of 23
elder abuse 45, 125–126
eldercide 67
Elementary School Guidance and Counseling 166–167
11 Myths of Media Violence, The (Potter) 92–93
emotional abuse 2
Encyclopaedia Britannica 174
Encyclopedia of Peace, Violence, and Conflict 62, 63
Entertainment Software Rating Board (ESRB) 159
environment and war 173
ESRB (Entertainment Software Rating Board) 159
ethnicity. *See* violence against populations
European Addiction Research 40
European Archives of Psychiatry and Clinical Neuroscience 84
European Psychiatry and Clinical Neuroscience 78
exercise 20–21, 51

F

fact v. fiction
  alcohol and violence 14
  bullying 23–24, 139

communities and violence 28
drugs and violence 38
family violence 41
gang violence 61
homicide 66
intermittent explosive disorder 79
media and violence 93
police officers 87
prevalence of violent crime 164
rehabilitation and treatment of
  perpetrators 129
suicide 136
violence, effects of 175–176
weapons of violence 179
workplace violence 186
Family Relations 19
family violence **41–47**
  about 7
  child abuse 41–42, 43
  cycles of violence 45–47
  discipline v. abuse 42–44
  elder abuse 45
  intergenerational transmission of
    violence 104–105
Federal Bureau of Investigation
(FBI)
  classes of violent crime 4, 31
  hate crimes 64
  homicide 66
  sexual violence 121
  terrorism 145, 150
Federal Trade Commission 159
felonies 32, 72
Fight Crime: Invest in Kids 25
fight or flight response **48–53**
  biological response 48
  enhancing your mood 50–52
  hardy personalities 49–50
*Final Report and Findings of the
  Safe School Initiative, The* 103
Franklin, Karen 63
Fur 158

G

gang violence **53–61**
  acceptance by a gang 55–56
  history of 53–54
  prevalence of 56–58, 102
  and schools 58–60
  and teenage violence 138
gender
  and bullying 23–25
  and gang violence 58
  and retaliatory violence 102–103,
    105
  and suicide 133
genetics 16, 164
genocide 157–158
Goldman, Linda 91–92
Government Accountability Office
  (GAO) 147–148
Grant, Marcus 16
Green, Donald 63
Groth, Nicholas 121, 125
gun use. *See* criminals and violent
  activity; school violence; weapons
  of violence

H

Haggerty, LaTanya 87
hallucinogens 37
hate crimes **61–65**. *See also* violence
  against populations
  about 7
  efforts against 65
  ethnicity and police officers
    87–88
  mentality behind 62–64
  victims of 64–65, 140–141
hazing 183–184
Health and Human Services, U.S.
  Department of 13, 41, 43
heart disease 18–19
Hilliard, Robert 63
Holocaust 157
homicide 4, **66–69**, 93

homosexuality. *See* hate crimes
hormones 15, 84, 167–170
Human Brain Mapping 163

I

Identity: An International Journal of Theory and Research 153
impulse control disorders 78–80
incarceration **70–78**
  costs of 128–129
  goals of 76–78
  history of 70–72
  laws about 33–34
  parole 98–100
  sentencing offenders 73–76
  treatment programs and 96–98
  types of prisons 72–73
infanticide 67
information warfare 147–149
inhalants 37
intergenerational transmission of violence 104–105
intermittent explosive disorder **78–85**
  causes 83–84
  and impulse control disorders 78–80
  and self-inflicted injuries 80–83
  treatment 84–85
International Association of Police Chiefs 89
International Journal of Offender Therapy and Comparative Criminology 95
intimate partner abuse 43–44
intravenous drug use 38

J

jail. *See* incarceration
Janjaweed 158
Jones, Jeff 111
Journal of Adolescent Research 162
Journal of Child and Adolescent Psychiatric Nursing 19
Journal of Children and Society 165
Journal of Clinical Psychiatry 80
Journal of Consulting and Clinical Psychology 44, 47, 85
Journal of Criminal Justice 87, 88, 93, 105
Journal of Drug Issues 36
Journal of Education 28, 47
Journal of Experimental Social Psychology 101, 159, 162
Journal of Family Issues 47, 102
Journal of Family Violence 104
Journal of Gang Research 59
Journal of Interpersonal Violence 95, 155
Journal of Moral Education 154
Journal of Occupational and Environmental Medicine 183
Journal of Pain The 21
Journal of Pediatric Psychology 101
Journal of Personality and Social Psychology 50, 103
Journal of Rational-Emotive & Cognitive-Behavioral Therapy 17
Journal of Research in Personality 161
Journal of Research on Crime and Delinquency 129
Journal of Social and Personal Relationships 104
Journal of Social Issues 152
Journal of the American Academy of Child and Adolescent Psychiatry 91, 150
Journal of the American College of Cardiology 19
Journal of the American Medical Association 139
Journal of Youth and Adolescence 105

Justice, U.S. Department of
  bullying 23
  communities and violence 28
  costs of violence 128
  hate crimes 61, 64
  intimate partner abuse 43–44
  legal interventions 85
  sexual violence 120
juvenile courts 35
Juvenile Justice Bulletin 53–54, 55

K
Keith, Michael 63
Kelling, George L. 86
Kentucky Corrections Division 95
King, Martin Luther, Jr. 156
King, Rodney 87
Klanwatch Intelligence Report 63
Klein, M. W. 56, 59

L
Labor Statistics, U.S. Department of
  183
labor unions 184
Law and Human Behavior 77
laws 32–34
legal interventions 85–89
LeMoncheck, Linda 124
Levin, Jack 62, 65
Lindquist, Scott 123
Litvak, Jorge 16
Living on the Razor's Edge (Selekman)
  117
Loss of the Assumptive World, The
  (Goldman) 91–92

M
Maddi, Salvatore 49–50
mandatory sentencing laws 33
manslaughter. *See* homicide
Massalit 158
Mayo Clinic 79
McDevitt, Jack 62

media and violence 7–8, **90–94,**
  110–111, 170
Media Psychology 160
mediation 114
medical costs of violence 128
Medical Journal of Australia 169
Men Who Rape (Groth) 121
Merck Manual of Medical Information
  52
Michigan Model for School Health
  Education 113
misdemeanors 32, 72
Monitoring the Future survey 36,
  168
mood-enhancing behaviors 50–52
MTV (Music Television) 29–30
murder. *See* homicide
Music Television (MTV) 29–30

N
narcotics 37
National Center for Injury Prevention
  and Control 141, 177–178
National Center for the Victims of
  Crime 14, 127
National Center on Elder Abuse 125
National Child Abuse and Data
  System (NCANDS) 42
National Counterterrorism Center,
  U.S. 145
National Crime Victimization Survey
  5–6, 13, 138
National Cyber Security Center
  (NCSC) 149
National Elder Law Network 125
National Fire Protection Association
  179
National Highway Traffic Safety
  Administration 13–14, 107
National Institute for Labor Relations
  Research 184
National Institute for Occupational
  Safety and Health 186

National Institute of Child Health and Human Development 23
National Institute of Justice 86
National Institute of Justice Journal 165
National Institute on Media and the Family 170
National School Safety Center 144
National Survey of Drug Use and Health 37
National Youth Gang Survey 57
National Youth Violence Prevention Resource Center 30
NCANDS (National Child Abuse and Data System) 42
NCSC (National Cyber Security Center) 149
negative reinforcement 117
neglect, child 43
negotiation 113–114
New England Journal of Medicine 110, 169
New Scientist 38
Nielsen Group 90
nuclear weapons 179–180

O

Odd Girl Out (Simmons) 24
Office of National Drug Control Policy 37, 130
Office of Personnel Management, U.S. 186–187
Oklahoma City bombing 6
Organizational Behavior and Human Decision Processes 101

P

pain, physical 21–22
parole 98–100. *See also* incarceration
Pediatrics 161
penitentiaries. *See* incarceration
Phi Delta Kappan 166
physical fights 178

police officers 85–89, 127
populations, violence against **152–158**
positive reinforcement 117
Potter, W. James 92–93
prejudice. *See* hate crimes; violence against populations
prevention strategies 29, 58–59, 112–116, 186–187. *See also* rehabilitation and treatment of perpetrators
prison. *See* incarceration
probation 34
Proceedings of the National Academy of Sciences 83
property crimes 4–5, 93, 140–141, 179
Psychiatria 28
Psychiatry 150
Psychiatry Research 80–83
Psychological Bulletin 14, 43
Psychology in Spain 96
Psychology of Addictive Behaviors 15, 96
Psychopharmacology 84
Psychosomatic Medicine 21
punishment for crimes 34–35. *See also* incarceration

Q

questions and answers
alcohol and violence 15
anger management 18–19, 20–21
communities and violence 30–31
drugs and violence 36–37
family violence 42
gang violence 60
homicide 67
incarceration 130
legal interventions 89
media and violence 90–91
revenge 103–104
self-mutilation 118
sexual harassment 185
sexual violence 119

suicide 133
teenage violence 141
video games 160, 163, 170
war 172

R

racial groups. *See* hate crimes;
  violence against populations
RAINN (Rape, Abuse & Incest
  National Network) 41
rape 4, 119, 121–124
Rape, Abuse & Incest National
  Network (RAINN) 41
Raundalen, Magne 173
recidivism. *See* rehabilitation and
  treatment of perpetrators
rehabilitation and treatment of
  perpetrators **94–100**. *See also*
  prevention strategies
  costs of 129–131
  influences on recidivism 94–95
  parole and community service
    98–100
  in prisons 96–98
  for self-mutilators 118–119
relapse prevention 98
relaxation techniques 20–21
repeat offenders 33–34
*Report from the Surgeon General on
  Youth Violence* 92
*Report on the Growth of Youth Gang
  Problems* 56
RETHINK 19
revenge, cycle of' **100–106**
risky business self-test 9–10
Rivers, Gayle 175
road rage 79, **106–108**
Russ, Robert 87

S

schizophrenia 21–22
school violence **109–116**
  contagious nature of 110–111
  fear of classmates 111

prevention strategies 112–116
  scope of 109–110
  signs of violent students 144
School Violence (Jones) 111
sedatives 37
Selekman, Matthew 117
self-determination theory 107
self-mutilation 80–83, **116–119**
sentencing offenders 73–76
September 11 attacks 150–151, 175,
  179
serotonin 15, 84, 167
sexual harassment 124–125, 183,
  184–185
Sexual Harassment, A Debate
  (LeMoncheck) 124
sexual orientation. *See* hate crimes;
  violence against populations
sexual violence **119–126**
  and alcohol 14
  in institutions 125–126
  rape 121–124, 138–139, 142
  sexual harassment 124–125, 183,
    184–185
  against transgendered people 154
Simmons, Rachel 24
Small Groups Research 20
social costs of violence **127–132**
  crime, costs of 95
  enforcement costs 127–128
  legal and rehabilitation costs
    128–131
  medical costs 128
  war, social costs of 173–174
Social Forces 157
Social Justice Research 101
*Social Psychiatry and Psychiatric
  Epidemiology* 106
Social Science Journal 107
social skills 8, 166–167
*Sourcebook of Criminal Justice
  Statistics 2005* 128, 132
spanking 43
Special Report on Youth Violence 141

Statistical Abstract of the United States 2009 67
statistics
  alcohol and violence 13
  bullying 23
  costs of violence 95, 127
  drug use 36
  family violence 42, 43, 44
  gun violence 176-177
  hate crimes 64
  homicide 66-67
  incarceration 71
  intermittent explosive disorder 79-80
  recidivism 97
  school violence 109-110, 115
  sexual violence 120, 121
  suicide 81-82, 133-134
  teenage violence 138
  terrorism 145-146
  victims of violence 6
Steinberg, Laurence 164-165, 177
steroids 39-40, 167-170
stimulants 37
stress. *See* fight or flight response
Studer, Jeannine 167
Sudan 158
suicide **132-137**
  and alcohol 14, 143
  causes of 132-133
  and children 28
  and drug use 38
  intervention 135
  prevalence of 81-82, 133-134
  signs of 136-137
Suicide and Life Threatening Behavior 165

T

Tattum, Delwyn 25
teens and violence **137-145**
  perpetrators of violence 141-144
  victims of violence 138-141
  weapons used by teens 177-178

teens speak
  bullying 25-26
  costs of violence 131
  drugs and violence 39, 143
  family violence 44-45
  gang violence 54-55
  rehabilitation 99-100
  school violence 111-112
  sexual violence 120
television. *See* media and violence
terrorism **145-151**
  bioterrorism 149-150
  cyberterrorism 147
  defined 145-147
  living with 150
  prevention of 147-149
  September 11 attacks 150-151
  and war 174-175
testosterone 167, 169
Texas Youth System 98
therapy 18-20, 96-98. *See also* rehabilitation and treatment of perpetrators
thinking errors 17-18
three strikes laws 33-34
Time 90
token economy 96
Treatment of Drug Offenders 130
treatment of perpetrators. *See* rehabilitation and treatment of perpetrators
truth-in-sentencing laws 32-33

U

Understanding and Managing Bullying (Tattum) 25
Understanding and Preventing Violence 127
Uniform Crime Reporting Program 31-32, 66, 140

V

victims of violence 5-7, 138-141
video games. *See* media and violence

video games and violence 158–163, 170–171
violence, forms of 2–3
violence, history of 3–4
violence against populations 152–158. *See also* hate crimes
  ethnicity and police officers 87–88
  genocide 157–158
  LGBT populations 154–155
  motivations for 152–154
  racial groups 155–157
Violence Prevention Institute 55
violent behavior, causes of **164–171**
  deficient social skills 166–167
  hereditary influences 164
  hormonal and biological influences 167–170
  learned/environmental influences 164–165
  psychological impairments 165–166
  societal influences 170–171

W

Walker, Michael 58
war **171–176**
  environmental costs 173
  family and social costs 173–174
  financial costs 172–173
  human life costs 174
  terrorism 174–175

War Against the Terrorists, The (Rivers) 175
War Finance 172
War on Labor and the Left ,The 184
Washington Post, The 172
Waves of Rancour (Hilliard & Keith) 63
weapons of violence **176–182**
  chemical and biological 181
  cutting objects 178–179
  fires and bombs 179–181
  guns 141, 142, 176–178
  physical fights 178
What Works in Reducing Young People's Involvement in Crime 96
WHO (World Health Organization) 5, 27, 29, 119, 145–146
workplace violence **182–187**
  harassment 184–185
  hazing 183–184
  prevention of 186–187
  unions and anger 184
World Health Organization (WHO) 5, 27, 29, 119, 145–146
World Report on Violence and Health (WHO) 27, 119

Y

Youth Risk Behavior Surveillance System 109–110, 134, 138, 139, 177

Z

Zhagawa 158